THE

Plant-Based

METABOLIC

Cancer Cookbook

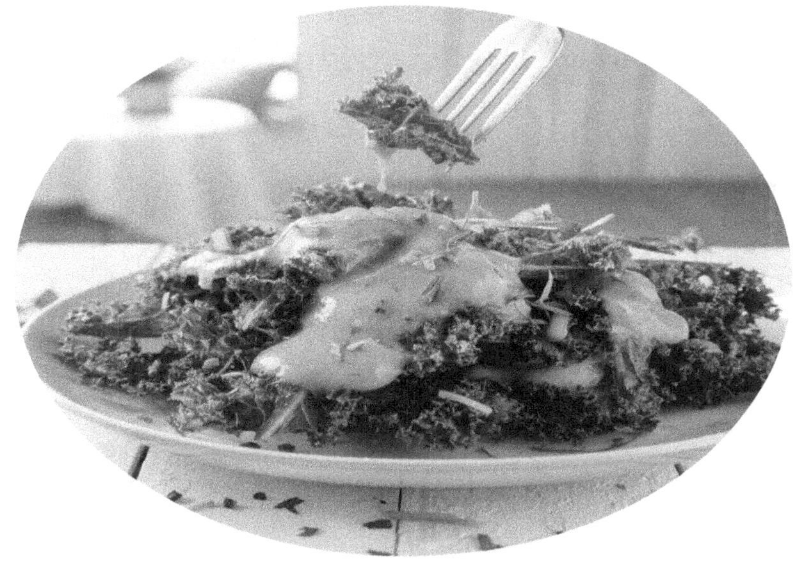

Science-Informed Recipes for Cancer Prevention and management

Kelley Hamilton

COPYRIGHT

© 2024 by Kelley Hamilton

Dedication

To all those who strive for a healthier tomorrow, May this book serve as a guiding light on your journey to wellness.

Table Of Contents

Surprise!

Dear reader, thank you so much for purchasing my book!

To make this book more (much more!) affordable, the images are all black & white, but I've created a special gift for you!

You can now have access, for FREE, to the PDF version of this book with the original images!

Keep in mind that some are originally black and white, but some are coloured

Go to page 96 and follow the instructions to download it.

I hope you enjoy it!

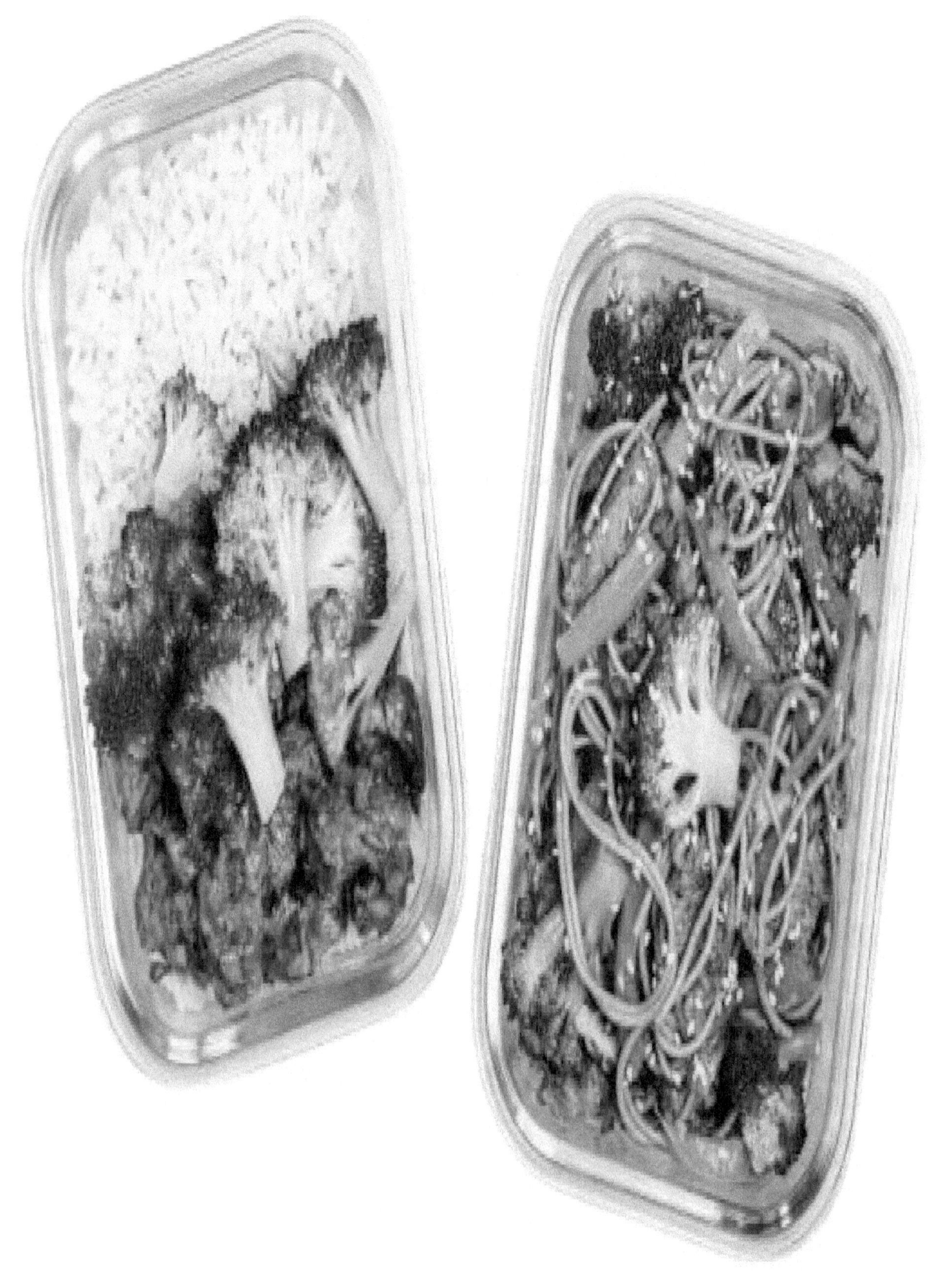

INTRODUCTION

It may be satisfying to follow an alkaline diet while traveling or eating out, and it is doable with the correct techniques. Maintaining your commitment to your health objectives while enjoying the trip may be achieved by accepting these circumstances with a proactive and adaptable mentality.

Make advance plans first. Do your homework before you go out to eat or book a vacation. Nowadays, a lot of eateries and vacation spots accommodate different dietary requirements, such as alkaline diets. To find eateries that provide food in keeping with alkaline principles, look up menus online. Many restaurants will fulfill special requests even if they don't specifically market alkaline choices. Never be afraid to give us a call in advance to ask about changes or substitutes. This method makes sure you have good selections and also gives you a sense of preparedness and confidence.

When eating out, concentrate on selecting wisely from the available selections. Choose mostly plant-based foods and ask to have them cooked with as little oil or salt as possible. For instance, a side order of grilled or boiled veggies may be a delicious accompaniment to a meal. Similarly, salads can be customized to your specifications by selecting a basic vinaigrette or requesting the dressing on the side. To keep track of what you're eating, don't be afraid to request sauces and dressings on the side or to swap out acidic for alkaline components when placing your order.

Although it takes a little more planning, traveling may be handled with little planning. Make sure you pack meals and snacks that fit your dietary requirements. When you're on the go, portable foods like raw nuts, seeds, fresh fruit, and veggie sticks work wonders to stave off hunger. To keep perishable goods fresh, think about purchasing an insulated bag or travel-friendly cooler. Make sure your food meets airport rules before you go, and if you want to keep hydrated, think about packing a reusable water bottle.

When planning lengthier vacations, consider the kinds of lodging you will choose. When you rent a property with a kitchen or kitchenette, you may cook for yourself and choose what items to use. It's common to be able to ask for a microwave or mini-fridge to assist with dinner preparation even while lodging in a hotel. This adaptability may be crucial to sustaining your nutritional objectives.

Eating at restaurants with a diverse clientele may be a rewarding experience. There are naturally alkaline alternatives in many cuisines. For instance, meals containing healthful grains, legumes, and fresh vegetables are common in Mediterranean cuisine. Asian food offers a wide range of rice and vegetable-based meals. Making your demands more precise and explicit may also be facilitated by becoming fluent in a few essential expressions linked to food preferences in the local tongue.

When there aren't many alkaline alternatives available, concentrate on the things you can manage. Select mostly plant-based meals, and when in doubt, request adjustments. Seize the chance to experiment with novel tastes and substances that complement the alkaline diet. Local markets and specialized shops often have fresh produce as well as substitute items that fit your diet.

Eating out or traveling requires some flexibility and patience to maintain an alkaline diet. It's important to keep in mind that straying from your ideal decisions sometimes is a normal part of the process. Take a balanced approach to these situations and concentrate on choosing the best course of action given the available options. Put your general health and well-being first, and understand that a bad meal or a bad day doesn't have to stop you from making progress.

In the end, being organized and making wise decisions are the keys to maintaining an alkaline diet while eating out or traveling. You may have fun without sacrificing your health objectives if you prepare ahead, communicate clearly, and have an optimistic outlook. Remember to be flexible and adaptable in your quest for an alkaline lifestyle, and embrace the adventure with confidence and inventiveness. You may improve your health and well-being with every step you take to follow your nutritional preferences.

Understanding the Connection Between Diet and Cancer

The connection between nutrition and cancer prevention has drawn more attention in recent years, especially in light of recent studies that demonstrate the potential effects of individual nutrients on cancer risk and prognosis. Particularly, plant-based foods have been central to this discussion, providing strong evidence that a diet high in fruits, vegetables, whole grains, and legumes may significantly lower the incidence of cancer and benefit people who are receiving treatment for the disease.

It has long been known from research that nutrition affects cancer risk via several different processes, such as cellular metabolism, oxidative stress, and inflammatory regulation. Foods based mostly on plants are rich in vital nutrients that promote these processes and may help prevent or treat cancer.

The abundance of antioxidants in plant-based diets is one of their main advantages. Free radicals are unstable chemicals that may cause oxidative stress and cellular damage. Antioxidants are substances that shield cells from these damages. The development of cancer is known to be influenced by this damage. Antioxidants are especially abundant in fruits and vegetables. Examples of these include berries, apples, and citrus fruits. These foods' antioxidants may aid in the neutralization of free radicals, decreasing oxidative stress and perhaps the risk of cancer.

, dietary fiber from plant-based diets has been associated with a decreased risk of many malignancies, including colon cancer. By encouraging regular bowel movements and fostering a healthy gut microbiota, fiber helps to maintain a healthy digestive system. This is important because inflammation and the metabolism of chemicals linked to cancer may be influenced by a healthy gut flora. Since obesity is a recognized risk factor for many cancers, high-fiber diets may also help control body weight, another significant factor in cancer risk.

Moreover, phytochemicals—naturally occurring substances found in plants—are essential in preventing cancer. For instance, studies have shown the anti-cancer effects of sulforaphane, which is present in cruciferous vegetables like broccoli and Brussels sprouts. It prevents the formation of cancer cells and aids in the body's detoxification of toxic chemicals. Similar to this, curcumin, the active ingredient in turmeric, has been the subject of much research due to its potential to reduce cancer cell growth and improve the efficacy of cancer therapies due to its anti-inflammatory and antioxidant qualities.

The significance of these nutrients derived from plants in the prevention and treatment of cancer is highlighted by recent studies. For example, research that was published in the Journal of the American Medical Association discovered a link between a decreased risk of cancer and larger intakes of fruits and vegetables. The American Journal of Clinical Nutrition published a thorough study that emphasized the benefits of plant-based diets in preventing various cancers, such as lung, prostate, and breast cancer. These studies support the notion that a diet high in plant-based foods may have a major impact on the prognosis of cancer.

Furthermore, the importance of nutrition in preventing cancer has been acknowledged by the World Health Organization (WHO) and other cancer research organizations. Red and processed meats have been categorized as probable carcinogens by the WHO's International Agency for Research on Cancer (IARC), which is in contrast to the finding that plant-based diets are positively associated with decreased cancer risk. This contrast with diets heavy on animal products emphasizes the potential advantages of plant-based diets in lowering cancer risk.

Plant-based diets are beneficial not just for preventing cancer but also for managing it after it has been discovered. Following a plant-based diet may help reduce the negative effects of cancer therapy, such as exhaustion, nausea, and appetite problems. Foods high in plant matter tend to be less inflammatory, which is good news for cancer patients since long-term inflammation may exacerbate the disease and worsen its adverse effects.

, plant-based diets may help with other health concerns that need to be managed during cancer treatment, such as keeping a healthy weight. Reducing treatment-related problems and increasing overall results require maintaining a healthy weight. Plant-based diets are rich in fiber, which increases satiety and may aid in better weight management.

Plant-based diets may provide psychological advantages in addition to physical ones. Many people take solace in the knowledge that they are actively managing their health, which may be powerful under difficult circumstances. Changing to a plant-based diet may also increase one's knowledge of and control over their health, which can improve their general well-being even more.

Overall, scientific evidence is supporting the link between diet and cancer more and more, with plant-based diets standing out as a particularly advantageous choice for managing and preventing cancer. Plant-based diets have a higher concentration of antioxidants, fiber, and phytochemicals, which help to prevent cancer. Furthermore, recent studies demonstrate the benefits of plant-based diets in lowering cancer risk and assisting those receiving treatment. A growing body of research indicates that including more plant-based foods in one's diet may significantly enhance health outcomes and successfully manage cancer.

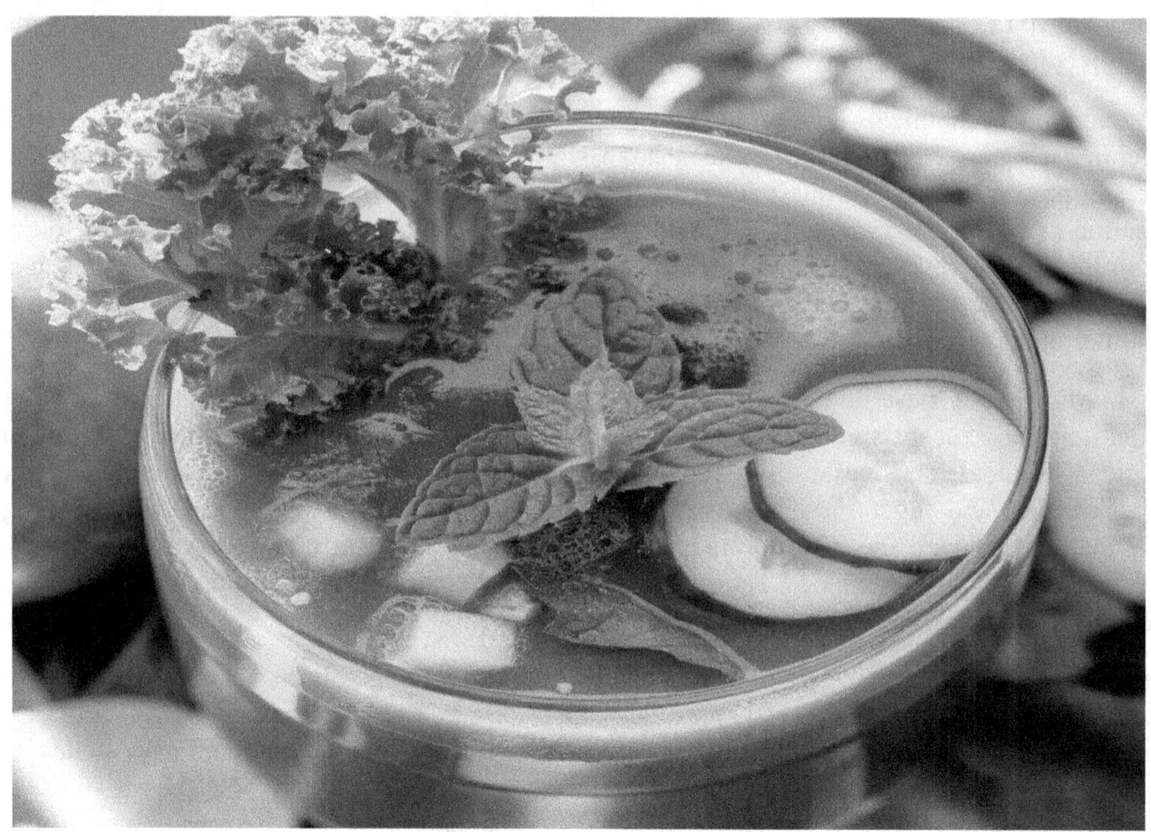

The Science Behind Plant-Based Nutrition

The foundation of plant-based nutrition is the emphasis on eating foods that come from plants, such as fruits, vegetables, whole grains, nuts, and seeds. This dietary strategy is unique in that it emphasizes plant foods that have been lightly or never processed, while avoiding or consuming less animal items. The fundamental tenets of plant-based nutrition center on giving the body the nutrients it needs while limiting its exposure to toxins that are often present in meals derived from animals.

Nutrient density is the central idea of plant-based nutrition. Plant-based diets are often low in calories and saturated fats but high in vitamins, minerals, and other healthful ingredients. For instance, leafy greens like kale and spinach are a great source of calcium and iron in addition to vitamins A, C, and K. Antioxidants, found in abundance in fruits like citrus and berries, protect cells from oxidative damage. B vitamins and fiber are found in whole grains like brown rice and quinoa. Nuts and seeds provide protein and good fats. The prevention of chronic illnesses and maintenance of general health depend heavily on this nutritional density.

The effect of plant-based diet on cancer-related metabolic pathways is one of its main features. The intricate web of chemical processes that the body goes through to stay alive is called metabolism. Plant-based diets have several positive effects on these processes.

First of all, dietary fiber, which is essential for controlling metabolism, is abundant in plant-based diets. Fiber facilitates regular bowel movements and improves digestion, both of which assist the body rid itself of possible carcinogens. Moreover, it promotes a healthy gut flora, which has been linked to decreased risk of cancer and inflammation. High-fiber diets have been shown in studies to help lower the risk of colorectal cancer by encouraging a healthy digestive system and shortening the amount of time that possible carcinogens remain in the colon.

Second, it has been shown that the phytochemicals included in plant-based diets have a positive effect on metabolic processes. Plants naturally contain substances called phytochemicals, which have been shown to have anti-cancer effects. For instance, the antioxidant and anti-inflammatory properties of flavonoids, which are present in fruits, vegetables, and tea, may lower the risk of cancer. Carotenoids, including beta-carotene, which is present in sweet potatoes and carrots, also support cellular health and may be able to stop the growth of cancer.

, plant-based diets assist in regulating blood sugar and insulin sensitivity. Elevated blood sugar and insulin resistance have been linked to an increased risk of many malignancies, including prostate and breast cancer. Because they are rich in fiber and low in refined carbohydrates, plant-based diets assist in stabilizing blood sugar levels and enhancing insulin sensitivity. Maintaining this equilibrium is essential for controlling current circumstances and lowering the risk of cancer.

Plant-based diets also affect inflammation, which is a major factor in the onset and spread of cancer. Because chronic inflammation encourages cellular damage and tumor development, it is associated with an increased risk of cancer. Foods derived from plants, which are high in anti-inflammatory substances, reduce this risk. For instance, it has been shown that the omega-3 fatty acids in walnuts and flaxseeds lower inflammation and promote general health. In a similar vein, the antioxidants included in plant-based diets aid in the reduction of oxidative stress and the neutralization of free radicals, therefore reducing inflammation.

Moving to a plant-based diet has many health advantages above just preventing cancer. The health of the heart is among the most important advantages. Diets focused mostly on plants are linked to lowered blood pressure, cholesterol, and heart disease risk. Plant foods have a high fiber content that aids in lowering LDL cholesterol, a key cause of cardiovascular disease. Furthermore, nuts and seeds' abundance of heart-healthy fats lowers inflammation and promotes cardiovascular health.

Another important advantage of a plant-based diet is weight control. When opposed to diets heavy in animal products, plant-based diets often include less calories and harmful fats. This may result in a healthy body weight and a lower chance of obesity-related diseases including diabetes and certain types of cancer. Plant-based meals include fiber, which helps people feel fuller for longer periods and consume fewer calories overall.

Eating a plant-based diet also helps to maintain metabolic health by improving blood sugar regulation. Many plant-based foods have a low glycemic index, which helps reduce the risk of insulin resistance and blood sugar rises. Those who already have diabetes or are at risk of getting it will benefit most from this since stable blood sugar levels improve metabolic health overall and lower the likelihood of complications.

, eating a plant-based diet helps to maintain better intestinal health. The high fiber content promotes a healthy gut flora and facilitates digestion, both of which are critical for the absorption of nutrients and general wellbeing. Preventing gastrointestinal problems, boosting immunity, and preserving energy levels all depend on a healthy digestive system.

Not to be overlooked is the effect plant-based nourishment has on the environment. A plant-based diet minimizes the negative environmental effects of animal husbandry, such as decreased water consumption, greenhouse gas emissions, and land degradation. This is in line with the increasing awareness of sustainability and the requirement of making ecologically friendly food choices.

, the foundation of plant-based nutrition is the consumption of foods high in nutrients that minimize the intake of toxic chemicals while offering vital vitamins, minerals, and therapeutic compounds. Plant-based diets have a substantial effect on cancer-related metabolic pathways, and there is evidence that they also help to reduce inflammation, control blood sugar, and improve digestive health. A plant-based diet has several health advantages, such as better blood sugar regulation, weight management, improved digestive health, and improved cardiovascular health. Adopting a plant-based diet is a comprehensive approach to well-being since it promotes environmental sustainability in addition to individual health.

How This Cookbook Can Support Your Journey

The foundation of plant-based nutrition is the emphasis on eating foods that come from plants, such as fruits, vegetables, whole grains, nuts, and seeds. This dietary strategy is unique in that it emphasizes plant foods that have been lightly or never processed while avoiding or consuming fewer animal items. The fundamental tenets of plant-based nutrition center on giving the body the nutrients it needs while limiting its exposure to toxins that are often present in meals derived from animals.

Nutrient density is the central idea of plant-based nutrition. Plant-based diets are often low in calories and saturated fats but high in vitamins, minerals, and other healthful ingredients. For instance, leafy greens like kale and spinach are a great source of calcium and iron in addition to vitamins A, C, and K. Antioxidants, found in abundance in fruits like citrus and berries, protect cells from oxidative damage. B vitamins and fiber are found in whole grains like brown rice and quinoa. Nuts and seeds provide protein and good fats. The prevention of chronic illnesses and maintenance of general health depend heavily on this nutritional density.

The effect of a plant-based diet on cancer-related metabolic pathways is one of its main features. The intricate web of chemical processes that the body goes through to stay alive is called metabolism. Plant-based diets have several positive effects on these processes.

First of all, dietary fiber, which is essential for controlling metabolism, is abundant in plant-based diets. Fiber facilitates regular bowel movements and improves digestion, both of which assist the body rid itself of possible carcinogens. Moreover, it promotes a healthy gut flora, which has been linked to decreased risk of cancer and inflammation. High-fiber diets have been shown in studies to help lower the risk of colorectal cancer by encouraging a healthy digestive system and shortening the amount of time that possible carcinogens remain in the colon.

Second, it has been shown that the phytochemicals included in plant-based diets have a positive effect on metabolic processes. Plants naturally contain substances called phytochemicals, which have been shown to have anti-cancer effects. For instance, the antioxidant and anti-inflammatory properties of flavonoids, which are present in fruits, vegetables, and tea, may lower the risk of cancer. Carotenoids, including beta-carotene, which is present in sweet potatoes and carrots, also support cellular health and may be able to stop the growth of cancer.

, plant-based diets assist in regulating blood sugar and insulin sensitivity. Elevated blood sugar and insulin resistance have been linked to an increased risk of many malignancies, including prostate and breast cancer. Because they are rich in fiber and low in refined carbohydrates, plant-based diets assist in stabilizing blood sugar levels and enhance insulin sensitivity. Maintaining this equilibrium is essential for controlling current circumstances and lowering the risk of cancer.

Plant-based diets also affect inflammation, which is a major factor in the onset and spread of cancer. Because chronic inflammation encourages cellular damage and tumor development, it is associated with an increased risk of cancer. Foods derived from plants, which are high in anti-inflammatory substances, reduce this risk. For instance, it has been shown that the omega-3 fatty acids in walnuts and flaxseeds lower inflammation and promote general health. In a similar vein, the antioxidants included in plant-based diets aid in the reduction of oxidative stress and the neutralization of free radicals, therefore reducing inflammation.

Moving to a plant-based diet has many health advantages above just preventing cancer. The health of the heart is among the most important advantages. Diets focused mostly on plants are linked to lowered blood pressure, cholesterol, and heart disease risk. Plant foods have a high fiber content that aids in lowering LDL cholesterol, a key cause of cardiovascular disease. Furthermore, nuts and seeds' abundance of heart-healthy fats lowers inflammation and promotes cardiovascular health.

Another important advantage of a plant-based diet is weight control. When opposed to diets heavy on animal products, plant-based diets often include fewer calories and harmful fats. This may result in a healthy body weight and a lower chance of obesity-related diseases including diabetes and certain types of cancer. Plant-based meals include fiber, which helps people feel fuller for longer periods and consume fewer calories overall.

Eating a plant-based diet also helps to maintain metabolic health by improving blood sugar regulation. Many plant-based foods have a low glycemic index, which helps reduce the risk of insulin resistance and blood sugar rises. Those who already have diabetes or are at risk of getting it will benefit most from this since stable blood sugar levels improve metabolic health overall and lower the likelihood of complications.

eating a plant-based diet helps to maintain better intestinal health. The high fiber content promotes healthy gut flora and facilitates digestion, both of which are critical for the absorption of nutrients and general well-being. Preventing gastrointestinal problems, boosting immunity, and preserving energy levels all depend on a healthy digestive system.

Not to be overlooked is the effect plant-based nourishment has on the environment. A plant-based diet minimizes the negative environmental effects of animal husbandry, such as decreased water consumption, greenhouse gas emissions, and land degradation. This is in line with the increasing awareness of sustainability and the requirement of making ecologically friendly food choices.

Tthe foundation of plant-based nutrition is the consumption of foods high in nutrients that minimize the intake of toxic chemicals while offering vital vitamins, minerals, and therapeutic compounds. Plant-based diets have a substantial effect on cancer-related metabolic pathways, and there is evidence that they also help to reduce inflammation, control blood sugar, and improve digestive health. A plant-based diet has several health advantages, such as better blood sugar regulation, weight management, improved digestive health, and improved cardiovascular health. Adopting a plant-based diet is a comprehensive approach to well-being since it promotes environmental sustainability in addition to individual health.

CHAPTER 1

The Fundamentals of a Plant-Based Diet

Consuming foods produced from plants, such as fruits, vegetables, whole grains, legumes, nuts, and seeds, is the main component of a plant-based diet. A plant-based diet mostly emphasizes plant foods but may sometimes contain minor quantities of animal goods, in contrast to veganism, which forbids all animal products. The fundamental idea is to base the majority of one's diet on plant-based foods since they are thought to provide a host of health advantages and enhance general well-being.

The focus on nutrient-dense foods that are high in vitamins, minerals, fiber, and antioxidants forms the foundation of a plant-based diet. This strategy promotes the consumption of a broad range of fruits and vegetables, which provide important nutrients and support a balanced diet. essential are whole grains like brown rice, quinoa, and oats, which provide vital elements including fiber, minerals, and B vitamins. A plant-based diet must include legumes since they are an excellent source of fiber and protein. Legumes include beans, lentils, and peas. Nuts and seeds, such as flaxseeds, chia seeds, and almonds, provide extra vitamins and minerals, protein, and good fats.

Foods that come from animals, such as meat, chicken, fish, dairy products, and eggs, are generally not allowed in a plant-based diet. Furthermore, because processed foods are incompatible with the principles of a plant-based diet, which emphasizes whole, unprocessed foods, processed foods rich in harmful fats and refined sugars are often avoided.

Making the switch to a plant-based diet may be a life-changing experience that calls for incremental adjustments rather than a drastic makeover. Increasing the number of plant-based meals you eat each week is a good place to start. This may include setting up certain days of the week as plant-based meals or trying out different plant-based dishes to discover which ones work best for your way of living. You may learn more about how plant-based foods influence your health and how to prepare them by progressively increasing the amount of plant-based meals you eat.

Finding plant-based substitutes for frequently used animal products is another crucial component of a seamless changeover. For example, plant-based cheeses and yogurts may be used instead of conventional dairy products, as can plant-based milk alternatives like almond or oat milk. When cooking, substitutes for meat, such as tofu or tempeh, may give the same texture and protein. You may ease the transition and make it more pleasurable by looking at these options.

Planning and preparing meals is another essential part of switching to a plant-based diet. Making a meal plan in advance helps you resist the need to turn to more convenient, animal-based foods by ensuring that you always have a range of nutrient-dense alternatives accessible. Meal preparation takes effort, but it may help you stick to a plant-based diet—especially if you have a hectic schedule. When you are short on time, making big quantities of plant-based recipes and freezing parts might be a useful alternative.

A major factor in facilitating a more seamless transition is education. Maintaining your health requires being aware of the nutritional requirements of a plant-based diet and making sure you are fulfilling them. The focus should be placed on the following essential nutrients: iron, which can be found in legumes and leafy greens; calcium, which can be found in fortified plant milk and leafy greens; omega-3 fatty acids, which can be found in flaxseeds, chia seeds, and walnuts; and vitamin B12, which is typically found in animal products and may require supplementation or fortified foods in a plant-based diet.

For those thinking about adopting a plant-based diet, common misunderstandings about it might sometimes provide difficulties. A common misconception is that diets based on plants are naturally low in protein. Many plant-based meals have a sufficient amount of protein, even while it's true that plant-based protein sources may not have the same amino acid profiles as animal products. Good sources of protein that may satisfy daily needs include quinoa, edamame, lentils, and chickpeas when included in a well-balanced diet.

There's also a misperception that plant-based diets are bland. As it happens, cooking with plants provides a wide variety of tastes and textures. Spices, herbs, and a variety of cooking methods may improve the flavor of plant-based foods, making them more gratifying and entertaining. There is something for every taste in plant-based food because of its versatility, which ranges from filling stews and aromatic curries to crisp salads and creative smoothies.

There's also a misconception that plant-based diets are costly or hard to stick to. It's not always expensive to follow a plant-based diet, even if certain specialized plant-based goods might be pricey. Budget-friendly staples like rice, beans, lentils, and seasonal vegetables may serve as the cornerstone of a well-balanced meal. You may control expenses and yet enjoy a wide range of delectable meals by emphasizing healthy foods and reducing processed foods.

Finally, some individuals believe that plant-based diets don't provide enough energy or support athletic performance. On the other hand, a lot of athletes do well on plant-based diets, showing that high energy and nutritional demands may be satisfied by eating plant-based meals. Athletes may follow a plant-based diet and yet attain peak performance and recovery with proper planning and an emphasis on foods high in nutrients.

A plant-based diet promotes the intake of foods originating from plants, which has many health advantages and enhances general well-being. To make the switch to this diet, one must gradually increase the amount of plant-based meals, look into substitutes for animal products, and concentrate on meal preparation and planning. Dispelling widespread myths may facilitate the shift and emphasize how varied, tasty, and nutrient-dense plant-based diets are. People may adopt a plant-based diet and get the many health advantages by learning the basics and taking proactive measures to overcome any obstacles.

Key Ingredients for Cancer Prevention

Certain plant-based substances are particularly effective in preventing cancer because of their unique qualities. By including these foods in your diet, you may lower your risk of cancer and proactively promote general health. These ingredients are high in fiber, phytonutrients, and antioxidants, all of which are vital for defending the body against cancer.

Free radicals are unstable chemicals that may cause oxidative damage to cells, which can result in cancer and other chronic illnesses. Antioxidants are substances that help neutralize free radicals. Antioxidants, which are abundant in plant-based foods, aid in preventing this damage and preserving the health of cells. Berries, including blueberries, strawberries, and raspberries, are rich in flavonoids and vitamin C, which are antioxidants. These antioxidants help the body's immune system, which is crucial for locating and eliminating cancer cells, in addition to shielding cells from harm.

The primary ingredient in turmeric, curcumin, is another potent antioxidant. Many studies have been conducted on curcumin's anti-cancer effects. It has been shown in several studies to limit the growth of cancer cells and help decrease inflammation, which plays a major role in the development of cancer. Including turmeric in your diet may enhance the taste of your food and help prevent cancer.

Another essential element in the fight against cancer is fiber. Dietary fiber, which is plentiful in whole grains, legumes, fruits, and vegetables, helps to maintain a healthy gut microbiota and encourages regular bowel movements, both of which are beneficial to digestive health. Diets rich in fiber have been linked to a decreased risk of colon cancer in particular, as well as other cancers. By lowering their interaction with the intestinal lining and removing possible carcinogens from the digestive system, fiber can lower the risk of cancer.

Phytonutrients are plant-based chemicals that provide substantial health advantages, including antioxidants and fiber. These include glucosinolates, flavonoids, and carotenoids, each of which has a unique method of preventing cancer. Research has shown the anti-cancer effects of carotenoids, such as beta-carotene, which is present in sweet potatoes and carrots. They aid in immune system support and cell damage prevention. In a similar vein, flavonoids, which are present in foods like citrus fruits, onions, and apples, have anti-inflammatory and antioxidant properties that lower the risk of cancer.

Another class of phytonutrients present in cruciferous vegetables such as kale, broccoli, and Brussels sprouts is called glucosinolates. It has been shown that these substances improve the body's detoxification mechanisms and stop the spread of cancer cells. The particular glucosinolate contained in broccoli, sulforaphane, is especially well-known for its ability to prevent cancer. It may lower the risk of some malignancies by aiding in the activation of enzymes that detoxify toxic chemicals.

Including adaptable components that combat cancer in your diet may provide continuous defense and assistance. Not only might some of these foods help prevent cancer, but they are also simple to include in a wide range of recipes. For example, allicin, a substance with anti-cancer and immune-boosting qualities, is found in garlic. In addition to improving taste, adding garlic to your food may help prevent cancer.

Another adaptable component with strong anti-cancer qualities is green tea. Green tea, which is high in catechins and especially epigallocatechin gallate (EGCG), has been shown to possess anti-inflammatory and antioxidant properties. Regular use of green tea has been shown to improve general health and lower the risk of many cancers.

Another important component with many health advantages is ginger. It has ingredients including gingerol, which has antioxidant and anti-inflammatory properties. By promoting digestive health and reducing inflammation, including ginger in your diet may help prevent cancer.

Nuts and seeds, including walnuts, flaxseeds, and almonds, are great providers of antioxidants, fiber, and good fats. , they contain a lot of phytosterols, which have been shown to improve general health and decrease cholesterol. Including nuts and seeds regularly may provide a nutrient-dense supplement to your diet that helps prevent cancer.

Leafy greens, like spinach, kale, and Swiss chard, are filled with vitamins, minerals, and phytonutrients. They are high in folate, which is needed for DNA repair and synthesis. Sufficient consumption of folate has been associated with a decreased risk of several types of cancer, which makes leafy greens an important part of your diet.

Lastly, since they are rich in protein and fiber, legumes like beans, lentils, and chickpeas are a mainstay of diets designed to ward against cancer. They contribute to the general prevention of cancer by providing vital nutrients and promoting intestinal health.

You may simply include these adaptable cancer-fighting items into your meals and snacks by having a range of them stocked in your kitchen. This strategy guarantees that you will always get the benefits of their preventive qualities and promotes a wholesome, pleasurable diet. Adopting these components into your regular diet may help you lower your risk of cancer and promote long-term health.

Tips for Shopping and Meal Planning

A successful plant-based diet relies heavily on efficient meal planning. It guarantees that you get the nourishment you need, but it also helps you keep organized, cut down on time, and avoid wasting food. Careful preparation, smart buying, and inventive food utilization are all components of a successful meal plan.

To effectively plan meals, one important tactic is to make a weekly menu including a range of plant-based meals. Start by choosing dishes that suit your dietary requirements and your taste. Think of serving a variety of recipes that use various plant-based products, such as fruits, vegetables, grains, and legumes. This diversity makes your meals interesting and guarantees that you get a wide range of nutrients. Make a schedule for your meals, ensuring that breakfast, lunch, supper, and snacks are all easily prepared for busy days.

After you've decided on your menu, make a thorough shopping list that includes all the items needed for the meals you've chosen. Grocery shopping might be more productive if your list is divided into sections, such as vegetables, grains, and pantry essentials. You may expedite your shopping experience and prevent going back through the store by organizing products into groups.

When procuring plant-based components, prioritize purchasing entire foods and minimally processed items. In general, whole foods—such as fresh produce, whole grains, and fruits—are more affordable and nutrient-dense than their processed plant-based counterparts. Shopping in bulk may also be a cost-effective tactic. To save costs and lessen packaging waste, buy essentials like rice, oats, beans, and lentils in bigger amounts. These products are often less expensive in bulk bins at grocery shops than in pre-packaged varieties.

Consider using the following advice to make grocery shopping simpler:

1. **Opt for Seasonal Produce:** This is because these fruits and vegetables are sometimes more reasonably priced and fresh. Plan your meals around the produce that is in season by looking through the flyers from your local grocery store or farmer's market.
2. **Purchase Frozen Fruits and Vegetables:** Frozen food is often just as nutrient-dense as fresh food, and it's a practical and affordable alternative. The nutritional content of frozen fruits and vegetables is typically preserved by flash-freezing them while they are at their best. They're also a fantastic choice for food that isn't in season.
3. **Make Use of Online Shopping:** A lot of grocery shops enable you to explore items and make your shopping list from the comfort of your home using their online shopping choices. You can prevent impulsive buys and save time by shopping online.
4. **Make a Weekly Meal Plan:** By organizing your meals, you can guarantee that you use ingredients effectively and lower the chance of food waste. To get the most out of your ingredients, pick ones that are adaptable and can be utilized in a variety of recipes.
5. **Create a Recipe Bank:** Gather your best plant-based recipes, which should be easy to create and use ingredients that are usually found in stores. Meal planning may be facilitated by having a go-to list of recipes that will help you avoid making last-minute decisions.

Some cost-effective suggestions for sourcing plant-based products are as follows:

1. **Choose Store Brands:** Store brands might provide comparable quality to recognized brands at a lower cost. For products like grains, spices, and canned beans, compare costs and choose store brands.
2. **Prepare for Leftovers:** Make bigger amounts of food and schedule the usage of leftovers for different meals throughout the week. By using this method, you may maximize the use of your components while cutting down on cooking time.
3. **Grow Your Herbs:** You may save money and have fresh ingredients for your meals by cultivating herbs like mint, cilantro, and basil at home. Herbs may flavor your food without costing more, and they are simple to cultivate on windowsills or little pots.
4. **Cook from Scratch:** It may be less expensive to prepare meals from scratch as opposed to purchasing prepackaged plant-based foods. Compared to store-bought alternatives, homemade soups, stews, and sauces are often less expensive and more healthful.
5. **Benefit from deals and Coupons:** Look for plant-based product deals, discounts, and coupons. Purchasing non-perishable goods in bulk during sales may result in long-term cost savings.
6. **Utilize Leftover Ingredients:** Find inventive ways to use the ingredients you currently own. To cut down on wasteful spending and minimize food waste, organize your meals around what you already have in your fridge and pantry.

By implementing these techniques into your daily routine, you may better control your plant-based diet. You can keep up a satisfying and healthy plant-based diet without going over budget by carefully planning your meals, purchasing wisely, and using money-saving advice. Not only can thoughtful meal planning and shopping techniques improve health, but they also facilitate and stabilize the transition to a plant-based diet.

Essential Kitchen Tools and Techniques

You can make the most of plant-based cooking by gaining proficiency in key methods and stocking your kitchen with the appropriate equipment. Knowing what to get and how to utilize kitchen utensils may be quite beneficial, whether you're just getting started or trying to set up your space for a plant-based diet.

To start, there are a few kitchen gadgets that are very helpful for making plant-based meals. A chef's knife of the highest quality is necessary. It makes it possible to cut, slice, and dice fruits, vegetables, and herbs precisely. Purchasing a knife that is balanced and sharp may increase the effectiveness and enjoyment of preparing meals. A cutting board is essential, in addition to a quality knife. Select one that is hygienic and long-lasting. While bamboo and wooden boards are common options, plastic boards are easier to clean, which is crucial for food safety.

Measurement spoons and glasses are also essential. Precise measures are essential for adhering to instructions and attaining uniform outcomes, especially in baking or creating sauces and dressings. You can make sure that your meals come out as planned by using measuring spoons and cups that are simple to use and properly marked.

An essential appliance for making smoothies, soups, sauces, and dips is a high-speed blender. Pureed soups, handmade nut butter, and creamy smoothies bursting with fruits and vegetables are just a few of the plant-based meals that often make up a plant-based diet. Purchasing a robust blender may simplify these chores and lead to a plethora of culinary opportunities.

And a food processor is quite helpful. It can chop, slice, shred, and combine different components swiftly. This adaptability is especially helpful when preparing foods that need a lot of preparation, like hummus, pesto, or vegetarian burgers. Meal preparation may be expedited by using a food processor, which can save time and effort.

A good nonstick skillet or sauté pan is necessary for cooking. Vegetables, grains, and lentils may be cooked easily with it without sticking or burning. It's also helpful to have a big pot on hand for stews, soups, and boiling grains. For plant-based cooking, which often involves one-pot dishes, a stockpot or Dutch oven may be very helpful.

Rinsing beans, draining pasta, and washing produce all need a colander. To guarantee effective drainage, a good colander should be robust and include tiny pores. In a similar vein, a fine mesh strainer works well for washing tiny grains, sifting dry materials, and straining liquids.

There are a few fundamental strategies for cooking plant-based foods that are worthwhile to learn. A basic cooking method is sautéing, which is heating food in a tiny quantity of oil over medium heat. This is the best way to cook veggies rapidly without sacrificing their taste or texture. To avoid burning, it's crucial to monitor the heat when sautéing and to stir often.

Another crucial method for preserving the nutrition and color of veggies is steaming. By placing a steamer basket inside a saucepan, vegetables may be cooked uniformly and their vitamins and minerals preserved by the steam that circulates them. Steaming works especially well for cooking veggies that are crisp-tender and delicate greens like spinach or kale.

Vegetables' inherent sweetness and complexity of taste are enhanced by roasting. Vegetables get a deep, savory taste and caramelize when they are baked in a dry heat environment. Root vegetables including sweet potatoes, carrots, and beets are especially good roasted. Vegetables may have a better taste and texture if they are tossed in a little oil and spice before roasting.

Grain bowls are a further skill to learn. Because of its versatility, grain bowls may be made with many types of grains, proteins, and vegetables. Cook a foundation of grains, such as farro, brown rice, or quinoa, first. Next, include sautéed or roasted veggies, a source of protein such as tofu or beans, and a tasty sauce or dressing. In addition to being wholesome, grain bowls may be tailored to suit a variety of tastes and preferences.

Keeping your kitchen organized and easily accessible is essential for supporting a plant-based diet. Organize your cupboard so that basic plant-based foods are easily accessible. Sort products into groups, such as grains, beans, and canned veggies, then label containers so you can easily see what's inside. Keeping your pantry neat and orderly can help you cook more efficiently and guarantee that you always have the necessary items on hand.

In the same way, set aside a space for your fresh vegetables. Vegetables and fruits should be kept accessible and visible in their storage. Produce waste may be avoided by keeping an eye on what you have and using transparent containers or open shelves.

In addition, purchasing high-quality storage containers is crucial to sticking to a plant-based diet. Grain, bean, and nut storage in airtight containers will keep them fresh and avoid spoiling. Different kinds of ingredients may be accommodated and portion management made easier with a range of container sizes.

Consider creating a workstation with your most frequently used kitchenware and utensils to expedite dinner preparation. You might use this area as a counter to store your measuring instruments, cutting board, and knives. Cooking may be more efficient and pleasurable when these supplies are readily available.

You should also think about putting in place a strategy for organizing and monitoring your meals. This might be a digital app or a physical planner that helps you keep track of your pantry inventory, plan your weekly dinners, and make shopping lists. By using this method, you may make the most of your components and maintain organization.

Plant-based meal preparation may be made more efficient and pleasurable by stocking your kitchen with the necessary appliances and learning basic cooking methods. Thoughtful organization and strategic planning are necessary when setting up your kitchen to accommodate a plant-based lifestyle. This may improve your cooking experience overall and help you meet your nutritional objectives. With the correct resources at your disposal, you may easily adopt a plant-based diet and cook delicious, wholesome dishes.

CHAPTER 2

Energizing Breakfasts

Eating a healthy breakfast is essential for maintaining energy levels and promoting general health in the morning. The Green Smoothie Power Bowl is one particularly notable choice. This colorful breakfast dish offers a nutrient-dense start to your day with spinach, kale, avocado, banana, and a dash of almond milk. The combination of leafy greens offers a significant amount of calcium, iron, and vitamins A and C—all necessary for lowering inflammation and maintaining a strong immune system. Avocados and bananas provide potassium and good fats, which are essential for cellular health and long-term energy. Together, these components support blood sugar regulation and provide a continuous supply of energy for the day. This smoothie bowl has ingredients that may help prevent cancer in addition to providing you with energy for the morning. Antioxidants and phytonutrients found in leafy greens help fight oxidative stress and lower the risk of cancer.

Berry with antioxidants Another great option for a cancer-fighting breakfast is oatmeal. Antioxidants such as vitamin C, anthocyanins, and flavonoids are abundant in berries, which include blueberries, strawberries, and raspberries. These antioxidants aid in the body's defense against free radicals, which might otherwise cause cellular damage and malignant growth. Because of its high fiber content, which facilitates digestion and supports gut health, oatmeal makes a great basis. By encouraging regular bowel movements and minimizing the amount of time carcinogens spend in the digestive system, fiber helps to reduce the risk of colorectal cancer. When you combine the fiber of oatmeal with these antioxidant-rich berries, you get a potent breakfast that promotes lifespan and general health.

Black bean and sweet potato breakfast Another wholesome choice is a burrito, which combines sweet potatoes and black beans in a tasty tortilla. Beta-carotene, which is abundant in sweet potatoes, is a precursor to vitamin A, which is well-known for its involvement in the immune system and eyesight maintenance. , beta-carotene has antioxidant qualities that lower the risk of cancer. Conversely, black beans include fiber and protein, both of which are essential for preserving muscle mass and promoting digestive health. When combined, these components provide a well-balanced meal that promotes metabolic health and aids in blood sugar regulation. Legumes, such as black beans, may assist in creating a sensation of fullness and maintaining energy levels throughout the day, which lowers the chance of unhealthy eating.

Another delicious breakfast option that mixes chia seeds with the freshness of seasonal fruits is Chia Seed Pudding with Fresh Fruit. Chia seeds are a nutritious powerhouse, including high levels of fiber, protein, and omega-3 fatty acids. Omega-3 fatty acids have been associated with a lower incidence of cancer and have anti-inflammatory qualities. Chia seed fiber promotes healthy digestion and helps keep blood sugar levels steady. This pudding becomes even more nourishing when it's mixed with fresh fruit, such as kiwis or berries. Fruits boost the meal's overall health benefits by providing extra vitamins, minerals, and antioxidants. A tasty and nutritious breakfast is created when the subtle taste of chia seeds is balanced by the fruit's inherent sweetness.

These breakfast alternatives include components that assist cancer prevention in addition to providing critical nutrients. Whole plant-based foods high in fiber, antioxidants, and healthy fats may help you make breakfasts that keep you energized and promote long-term health. By guaranteeing that you begin the day with a nutritious edge that supports both your immediate energy demands and your general well-being, these meals help establish a favorable tone for the rest of the day.

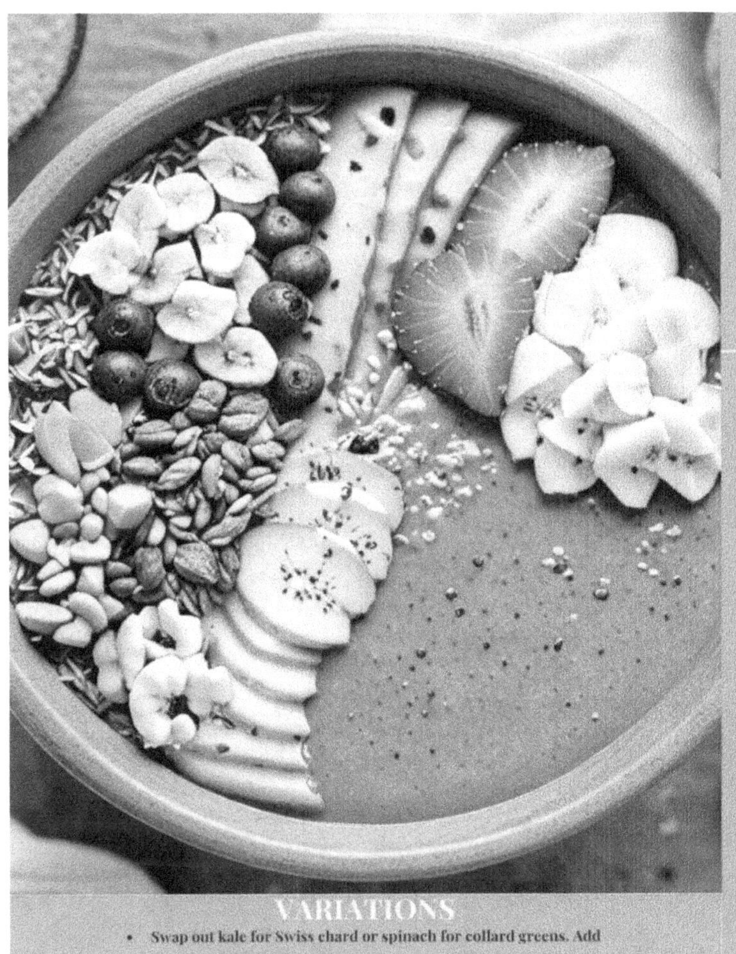

Green Smoothie Power Bowl

Prep Time
10 minutes

Cook Time
0 minutes

INGREDIENTS

- 1 cup fresh spinach
- 1 cup kale, stems removed
- 1 banana
- 1/2 avocado
- 1/2 cup unsweetened almond milk (or any plant-based milk)
- 1 tablespoon chia seeds
- 1 tablespoon hemp seeds
- 1 tablespoon almond butter
- Optional toppings: sliced almonds, fresh berries, coconut flakes, granola

VARIATIONS
- Swap out kale for Swiss chard or spinach for collard greens. Add a scoop of protein powder for an extra protein boost. For a sweeter smoothie, include a date or a splash of maple syrup.

DIRECTIONS

1. Prepare the Greens: Rinse spinach and kale thoroughly. Remove the stems from the kale.
2. Blend the Base: In a blender, combine spinach, kale, banana, avocado, and almond milk. Blend until smooth and creamy.
3. Add Seeds: Stir in chia seeds and hemp seeds. Blend briefly to combine.
4. Serve: Pour the smoothie into a bowl. Top with almond butter, and any of the optional toppings like sliced almonds, fresh berries, coconut flakes, or granola.

350 calories per serving, 10g protein, 20g fat, 35g carbohydrates, 8g fiber

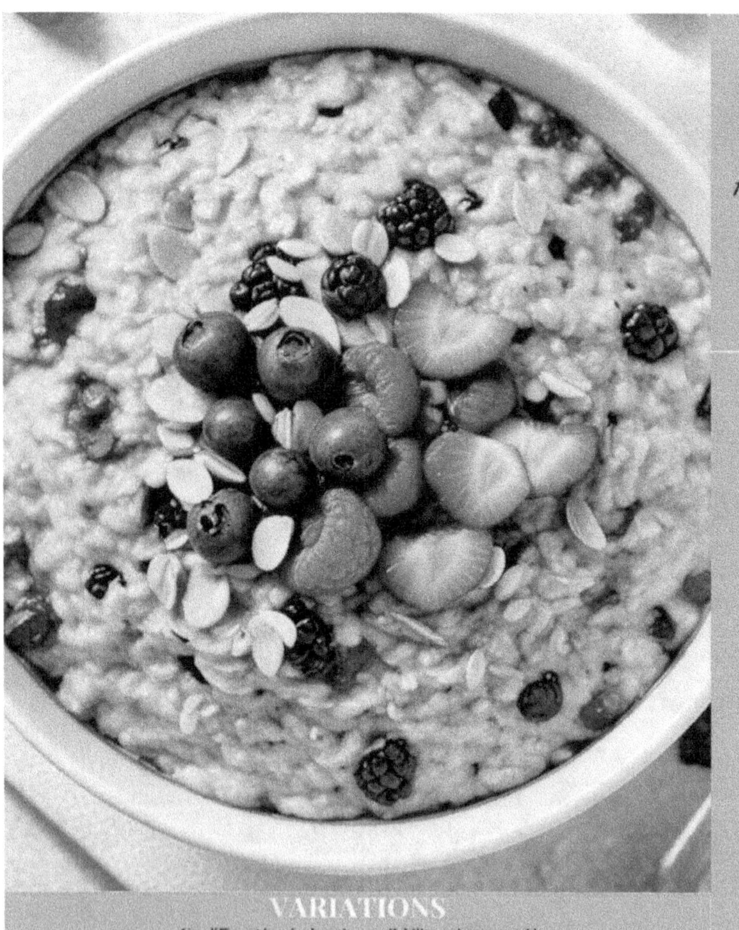

★★★★☆

Antioxidant Berry Oatmeal

Prep Time
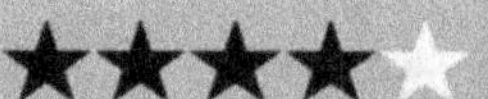
5 minutes

Cook Time
7 minutes

INGREDIENTS

- 1 cup rolled oats
- 2 cups water or plant-based milk
- 1/2 cup mixed berries (blueberries, strawberries, raspberries)
- 1 tablespoon chia seeds
- 1 tablespoon flaxseeds
- 1 tablespoon honey or maple syrup (optional)
- 1/2 teaspoon vanilla extract (optional)

VARIATIONS

Use different berries based on availability and season. Add nuts like walnuts or almonds for extra crunch and protein. For a creamier texture, stir in a spoonful of almond butter or coconut yogurt.

DIRECTIONS

1. Cook the Oats: In a medium saucepan, bring water or plant-based milk to a boil. Add rolled oats and reduce heat to a simmer. Cook for 5-7 minutes, stirring occasionally.
2. Prepare the Berries: While the oats cook, rinse the berries and slice any large ones like strawberries.
3. Combine Ingredients: Once the oats are cooked, stir in chia seeds, flaxseeds, honey or maple syrup, and vanilla extract if using.
4. Serve: Spoon the oatmeal into bowls and top with fresh berries.

300 calories per serving, 8g protein, 8g fat, 50g carbohydrates, 10g fiber

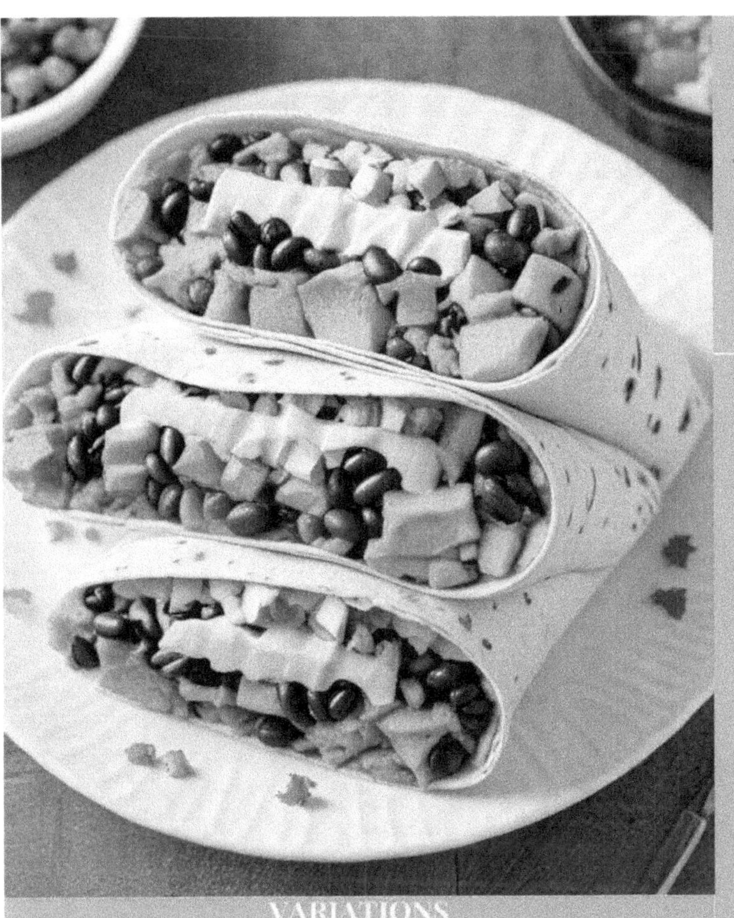

★★★★☆

INGREDIENTS

- 1 large sweet potato, peeled and diced
- 1 cup black beans, drained and rinsed
- 1/2 red bell pepper, diced
- 1/4 cup red onion, finely chopped
- 1 tablespoon olive oil
- 1 teaspoon cumin
- 1/2 teaspoon paprika
- Salt and pepper to taste
- 2 whole wheat tortillas
- Optional toppings: avocado slices, salsa, cilantro

VARIATIONS

For a spicier burrito, add diced jalapeños or a sprinkle of hot sauce. Substitute sweet potatoes with roasted butternut squash for a different flavor profile. You can also add a handful of spinach or kale for extra greens.

DIRECTIONS

1. Cook the Sweet Potato: Heat olive oil in a skillet over medium heat. Add diced sweet potato and cook for 10-12 minutes, stirring occasionally, until tender.
2. Add Vegetables: Stir in the red bell pepper and red onion. Cook for an additional 3-4 minutes.
3. Season and Mix: Add black beans, cumin, paprika, salt, and pepper. Cook for another 2-3 minutes, until beans are heated through and flavors are well combined.
4. Assemble the Burritos: Warm the tortillas in a separate pan or microwave. Spoon the sweet potato and black bean mixture onto each tortilla. Add any optional toppings such as avocado slices, salsa, or cilantro. Roll up the tortillas to enclose the filling.

400 calories per serving, 15g protein, 10g fat, 60g carbohydrates, 12g fiber

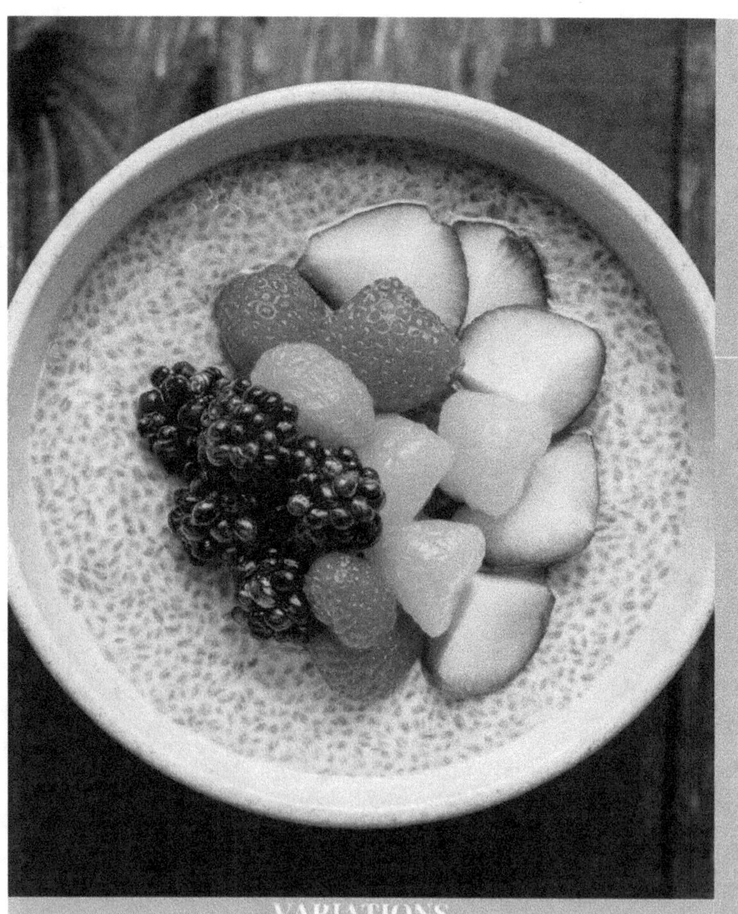

Chia Seed Pudding with Fresh Fruit

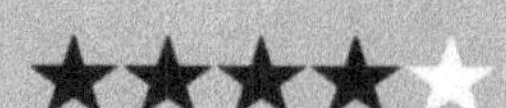

Prep Time

5 minutes

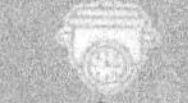

Cook Time

0 minutes

INGREDIENTS

- 1/4 cup chia seeds
- 1 cup unsweetened almond milk (or any plant-based milk)
- 1 tablespoon maple syrup or honey
- 1/2 teaspoon vanilla extract
- 1/2 cup fresh fruit (berries, kiwi, mango, etc.)

VARIATIONS

Experiment with different plant-based milks such as coconut or oat milk. Add spices like cinnamon or nutmeg for extra flavor. For a richer pudding, stir in a spoonful of almond butter or coconut yogurt.

DIRECTIONS

1. Mix the Pudding: In a bowl, combine chia seeds, almond milk, maple syrup, and vanilla extract. Stir well to ensure chia seeds are evenly distributed.
2. Refrigerate: Cover the bowl and refrigerate for at least 4 hours or overnight to allow the chia seeds to absorb the liquid and form a gel-like consistency.
3. Serve: Spoon the chia pudding into bowls or glasses. Top with fresh fruit of your choice.

250 calories per serving, 7g protein, 12g fat, 30g carbohydrates, 10g fiber

CHAPTER 3

Nutrient-Rich Lunches

A tasty and nutritious lunch choice that is high in nutrients and taste is quinoa and roasted veggie salad. Packed full of nutrients, quinoa is a complete protein source that includes all nine necessary amino acids. This makes it a great option for anyone who wants to be sure they're getting enough protein while on a plant-based diet. Quinoa also has high levels of iron, magnesium, B vitamins, and fiber, all of which are beneficial to general health and may help prevent or treat cancer. Its high fiber content aids in blood sugar regulation and proper digestion, both of which are critical for sustaining a balanced diet.

When it comes to preparing vegetables, roasting improves their taste and nutritional value. Vegetables' natural sugars are caramelized during the roasting process, giving them a richer, deeper flavor. , this technique helps to retain the vitamins and minerals in the veggies more effectively than boiling, which may result in a considerable loss of nutrients. High-temperature roasting is a healthy cooking method because it may enhance tastes and provide a crispy texture without using a lot of fats or oils.

Another great option for a nutrient-rich lunch is a soup made with lentils and spinach. A well-balanced diet that combats cancer should include lentils since they are a great source of protein, fiber, iron, and folate. Their high protein content maintains muscular health and normal body processes, while their high fiber content facilitates digestion and lowers cholesterol. Lentils include iron which helps prevent anemia and folate which promotes cellular health, both of which are critical for avoiding cancer.

Lentils and spinach have synergistic effects when combined. Vitamins A, C, and K, as well as antioxidants like lutein and beta-carotene, are abundant in spinach. These nutrients support healthy skin, strong bones, and a functioning immune system. Spinach contains antioxidants that help fight oxidative stress and inflammation, two factors associated with the development of cancer. Spinach's strong iron concentration balances the iron in lentils, enhancing total nutrient absorption, and its high vitamin K content promotes good blood coagulation and bone health.

A tasty and nutritious choice that is filling and high in nutrients is the Mediterranean chickpea wrap. Plant-based protein, fiber, and a variety of vitamins and minerals, such as phosphorus, manganese, and folate, may all be found in plenty in chickpeas. Their high fiber content promotes healthy digestion and helps to keep blood sugar levels steady. Furthermore, substances including phytates and saponins, which have been shown to have anticancer effects, are present in chickpeas.

Antioxidants and healthy fats abound in Mediterranean foods including avocados, tomatoes, cucumbers, and olives. A mainstay of the Mediterranean diet, olive oil has anti-inflammatory qualities and is rich in heart-healthy monounsaturated fats. Lycopene, an antioxidant associated with a lower risk of cancer, is found in tomatoes, while avocados provide the wrap healthful fats and vitamins. These substances work together to promote general well-being and provide a host of health advantages.

A colorful and cooling choice, raw rainbow vegetable noodle salad emphasizes the advantages of eating raw veggies. Compared to cooked veggies, raw vegetables retain more of their vitamins and minerals since cooking may lead to some nutritional loss. Consuming an assortment of uncooked veggies offers an abundance of antioxidants, dietary fiber, and vital vitamins that promote general well-being and ward against cancer. This salad's vibrant assortment of veggies guarantees a wide variety of nutrients, such as potassium, folate, and vitamins A and C.

There are several benefits to switching from standard pasta to vegetarian noodles. Vegetable noodles are a lighter option yet have a pleasing texture and taste since they have fewer calories and carbs. They also include a lot of vitamins and fiber, which is good for your health. Incorporating a range of sauces and toppings to cater to diverse palates, vegetable noodles provide a crisp and vibrant touch to salads. This method promotes an eating plan high in nutrients that prevents cancer and helps you eat more veggies.

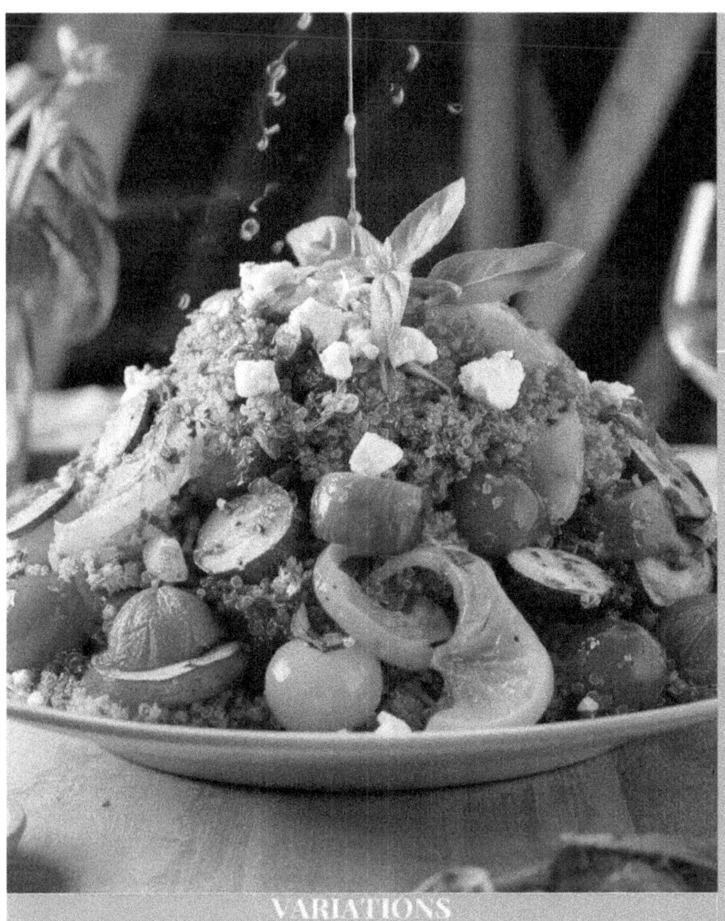

Quinoa and Roasted Vegetable Salad

Prep Time	Cook Time
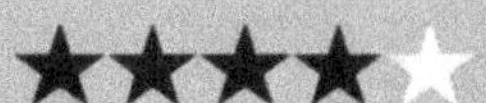	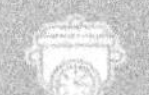
15 minutes	30 minutes

INGREDIENTS

- 1 cup quinoa
- 2 cups water
- 1 red bell pepper, diced
- 1 zucchini, sliced
- 1 cup cherry tomatoes, halved
- 1 red onion, diced
- 2 tablespoons olive oil
- 1 teaspoon dried oregano
- 1 teaspoon paprika
- Salt and pepper to taste
- 1/4 cup crumbled feta cheese (optional)
- 2 tablespoons balsamic vinaigrette

VARIATIONS

Substitute quinoa with farro or bulgur for a different grain texture. Add fresh herbs like parsley or basil for added flavor. For a vegan version, omit the feta cheese.

DIRECTIONS

1. Cook Quinoa: Rinse quinoa under cold water. In a medium saucepan, combine quinoa and water. Bring to a boil, then reduce heat to low, cover, and simmer for 15 minutes. Remove from heat and let it sit, covered, for 5 minutes. Fluff with a fork and let cool.
2. Roast Vegetables: Preheat the oven to 400°F (200°C). On a baking sheet, toss red bell pepper, zucchini, cherry tomatoes, and red onion with olive oil, dried oregano, paprika, salt, and pepper. Roast for 20-25 minutes, or until vegetables are tender and slightly charred.
3. Combine Ingredients: In a large bowl, combine the cooked quinoa with roasted vegetables. Add crumbled feta cheese, if using, and drizzle with balsamic vinaigrette. Toss gently to combine.

350 calories per serving, 12g protein, 15g fat, 45g carbohydrates, 8g fiber

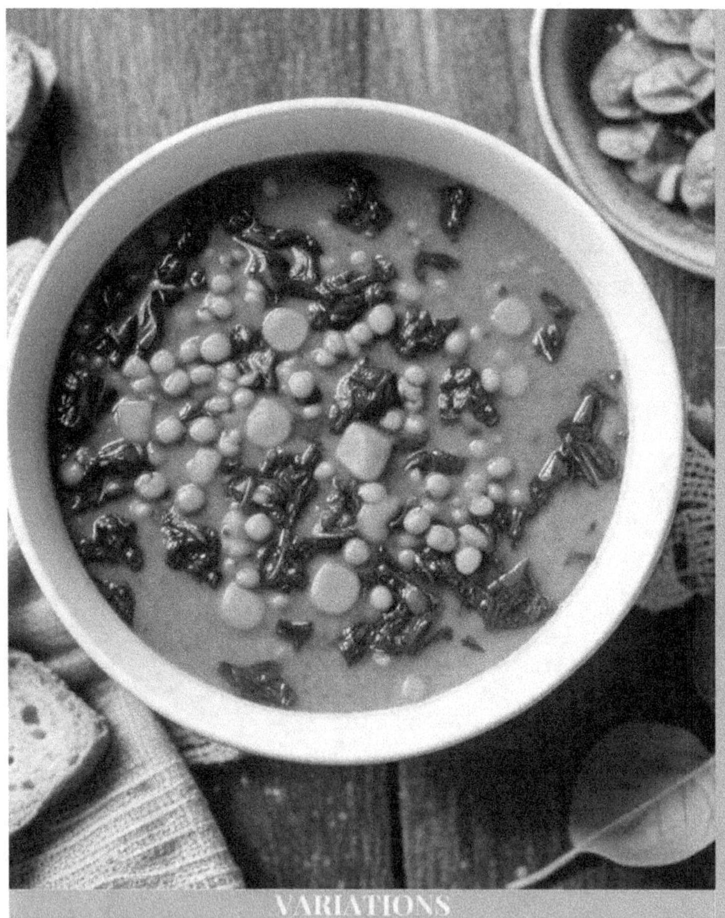

Lentil and Spinach Soup

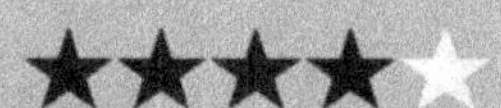

Prep Time

15 minutes

Cook Time

35 minutes

INGREDIENTS

- 1 cup dried green or brown lentils
- 6 cups vegetable broth
- 1 cup diced carrots
- 1 cup diced celery
- 1 onion, chopped
- 3 cloves garlic, minced
- 2 cups fresh spinach, chopped
- 1 teaspoon ground cumin
- 1/2 teaspoon turmeric
- 1/2 teaspoon thyme
- Salt and pepper to taste
- 1 tablespoon olive oil

VARIATIONS

Add diced tomatoes or a splash of lemon juice for extra flavor.
Substitute spinach with kale or Swiss chard. For a creamier texture,
blend part of the soup.

DIRECTIONS

1. Prepare Lentils: Rinse lentils under cold water and set aside.
2. Sauté Vegetables: In a large pot, heat olive oil over medium heat. Add onion, carrots, and celery. Cook for 5-7 minutes, or until vegetables are softened. Stir in garlic and cook for another minute.
3. Cook Soup: Add lentils, vegetable broth, cumin, turmeric, thyme, salt, and pepper. Bring to a boil, then reduce heat and simmer for 25-30 minutes, or until lentils are tender.
4. Add Spinach: Stir in chopped spinach and cook for an additional 5 minutes until spinach is wilted and tender. Adjust seasoning as needed.

250 calories per serving, 15g protein, 4g fat, 40g carbohydrates, 12g fiber

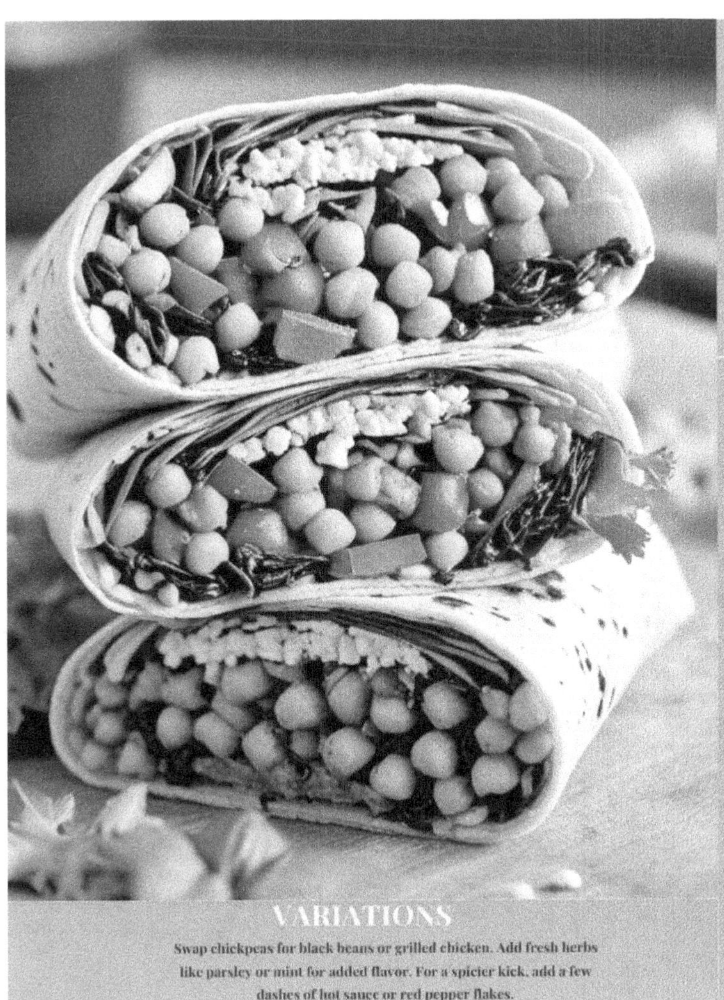

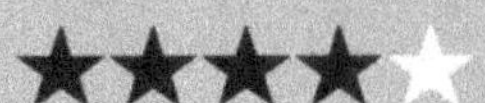

★★★★☆

Mediterranean Chickpea Wrap

Prep Time

10 minutes

Cook Time

0 minutes

INGREDIENTS

- 1 can chickpeas, drained and rinsed
- 1/2 cup diced cucumbers
- 1/2 cup halved cherry tomatoes
- 1/4 cup diced red onion
- 1/4 cup sliced Kalamata olives
- 1/4 cup crumbled feta cheese (optional)
- 2 whole wheat tortillas
- 2 tablespoons hummus
- 2 tablespoons tzatziki sauce (optional)

VARIATIONS

Swap chickpeas for black beans or grilled chicken. Add fresh herbs like parsley or mint for added flavor. For a spicier kick, add a few dashes of hot sauce or red pepper flakes.

DIRECTIONS

1. Prepare Filling: In a bowl, combine chickpeas, cucumbers, cherry tomatoes, red onion, olives, and feta cheese if using. Mix well.
2. Assemble Wraps: Spread hummus evenly over each tortilla. Spoon the chickpea mixture onto the center of each tortilla. Add tzatziki sauce if desired. Fold the sides of the tortilla over the filling and roll up tightly.
3. Serve: Cut wraps in half and serve immediately, or wrap in foil for an on-the-go meal.

400 calories per wrap, 15g protein, 12g fat, 50g carbohydrates, 10g fiber

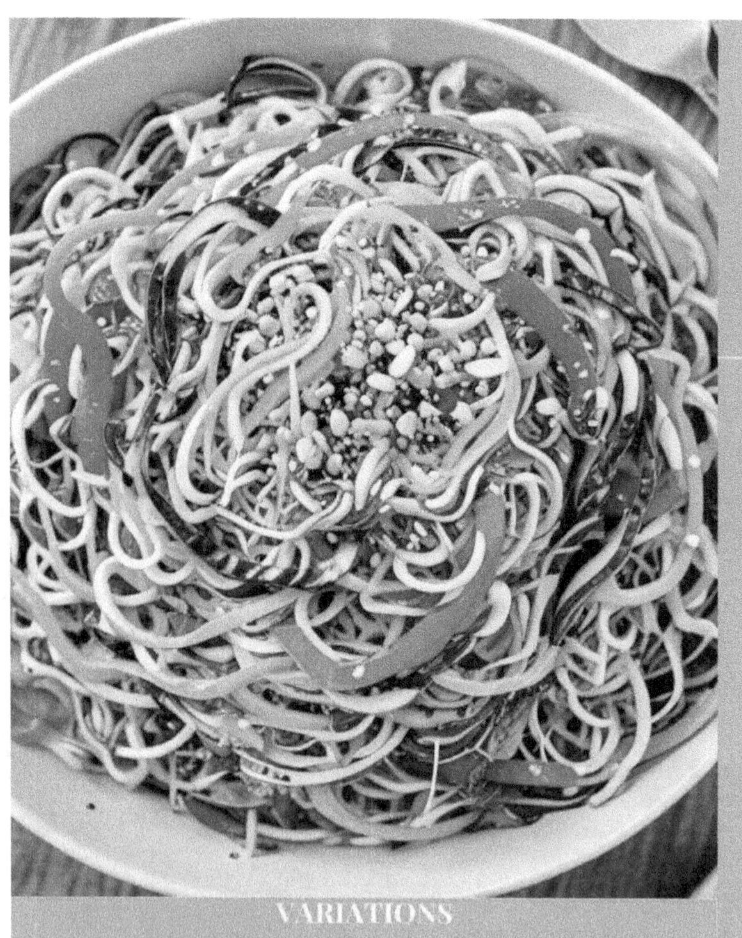

Raw Rainbow Vegetable Noodle Salad

Prep Time 
15 minutes

Cook Time
0 minutes

INGREDIENTS

- 1 large carrot, peeled and spiralized
- 1 zucchini, spiralized
- 1 red bell pepper, thinly sliced
- 1 cup cherry tomatoes, halved
- 1/2 cup red cabbage, shredded
- 1/4 cup fresh cilantro, chopped
- 2 tablespoons sesame seeds
- 3 tablespoons lemon juice
- 2 tablespoons tahini
- 1 tablespoon maple syrup
- 1 clove garlic, minced
- Salt and pepper to taste

VARIATIONS

Use different vegetables like cucumber or bell peppers for variety. Add avocado or tofu for extra protein. For a tangier flavor, substitute lemon juice with lime juice.

DIRECTIONS

1. Prepare Vegetables: Spiralize the carrot and zucchini. Thinly slice red bell pepper and halve cherry tomatoes. Shred red cabbage and chop cilantro.
2. Make Dressing: In a small bowl, whisk together lemon juice, tahini, maple syrup, garlic, salt, and pepper until smooth.
3. Combine Salad: In a large bowl, toss all vegetables with the dressing. Sprinkle with sesame seeds and chopped cilantro before serving.

200 calories per serving, 5g protein, 12g fat, 20g carbohydrates, 7g fiber

CHAPTER 4

Wholesome Dinners

A tasty and wholesome substitute for regular pasta is spaghetti squash with tomato basil sauce. When prepared properly, spaghetti squash has a stringy texture similar to pasta, which makes it a popular low-calorie alternative. This vegetable offers many health advantages since it is high in potassium, fiber, vitamins A and C, and all three. It's a great option for anyone trying to control their weight and maintain general health because of its high fiber content and low-calorie count. You may increase your intake of vital nutrients and lower your carbohydrate load by substituting spaghetti squash for conventional pasta.

One of the sauce's main ingredients, tomatoes is renowned for their ability to prevent cancer. They contain lycopene, a potent antioxidant associated with a lower risk of prostate cancer and other malignancies. Lycopene fights inflammation and oxidative stress, two factors that are known to contribute to the development of cancer. The herb used to season the sauce, basil, has many health advantages of its own. Flavonoids and eugenol are among the substances it contains that have antioxidant and anti-inflammatory properties. Tomatoes and basil work together to improve the dish's taste while offering strong protection against oxidative damage.

A plant-based, cancer-prevention diet would benefit greatly from the hearty and satisfying supper choice that filled bell peppers and cauliflower rice provide. A wonderful low-carb alternative to regular rice is cauliflower rice, which is created by shredding or processing cauliflower into a texture similar to rice. It has high levels of antioxidants, fiber, and vitamins C and K, all of which promote general health and help prevent cancer. Sulforaphane, one of the chemicals found in cauliflower, has been shown to have anti-cancer effects by aiding in detoxification and guarding against cellular damage.

Bell peppers that have been stuffed are not only filling but also adaptable and flexible. The bell peppers themselves are an excellent source of carotenoids, antioxidants, and vitamins A and C. These nutrients aid in oxidative stress reduction and immune system augmentation. The savory pepper filling and nutrient-dense cauliflower rice combine to provide a well-balanced meal that promotes health and satisfaction. Legumes, grains, and veggies are just a few of the contents that may be added to the meal to suit a wide range of palates and nutritional requirements.

A dish that is high in protein and may help prevent cancer is tofu stir-fried with broccoli and cashews. Soybeans are used to make tofu, which is a great plant-based protein source that is rich in essential amino acids and low in saturated fat. Isoflavones found in soy products, such as tofu, especially genistein, and daidzein, have been investigated for possible cancer-prevention properties. These substances can control hormone levels and guard against malignancies linked to hormones.

One of the main ingredients in the stir-fry, broccoli, is well known for its ability to prevent cancer. It contains a lot of sulforaphane, a substance that has been shown to improve detoxification and shield cells from harm. In addition, broccoli has a high content of antioxidants, fiber, and vitamins C and K, all of which support a strong immune system and may help reduce the risk of cancer. Cashews provide healthful fats, protein, and important minerals like zinc and magnesium. They are added to the stir-fry for crunch and taste. These nutrients promote heart health and enhance general health.

A tasty and nutritious supper option, sweet and spicy butternut squash curry mixes the natural sweetness of butternut squash with a mixture of fragrant spices. In addition to being tasty, butternut squash is a great source of fiber, potassium, and vitamins A and C. Because it contains a significant amount of beta-carotene, a type of vitamin A, it helps healthy skin, immune system, and eyesight. Butternut squash's fiber promotes healthy weight maintenance and helps with digestion.

Curry's seasonings, which include cinnamon, ginger, and turmeric, have many health advantages. Curcumin, a substance with potent anti-inflammatory and antioxidant qualities, is found in turmeric. The potential of curcumin to suppress the proliferation of cancer cells and improve the efficacy of traditional therapies has been investigated. having anti-inflammatory qualities, ginger and cinnamon may aid with blood sugar regulation and digestion. These spices work together to improve the curry's taste while also offering health advantages that help prevent cancer and promote general well-being.

These filling meals are full of nutrition and taste, so they're a great option for anybody trying to keep a balanced and healthful diet. These dishes enhance general health and prevent cancer by combining a variety of vegetables, healthy grains, and plant-based proteins with flavor and nutritional benefits.

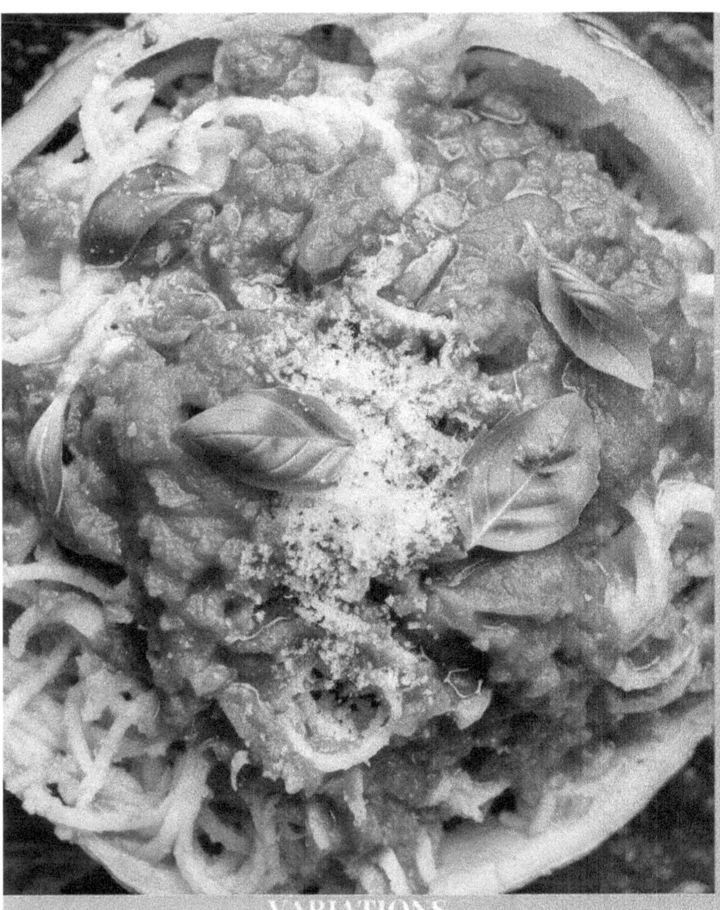

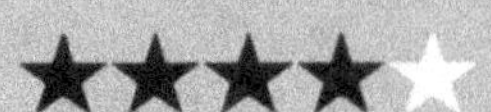

Spaghetti Squash with Tomato Basil Sauce

Prep Time	Cook Time
15 minutes	45 minutes

INGREDIENTS

- 1 medium spaghetti squash
- 2 tablespoons olive oil
- 1 onion, finely chopped
- 3 cloves garlic, minced
- 1 can (14.5 oz) diced tomatoes
- 1/4 cup tomato paste
- 1 teaspoon dried basil
- 1/2 teaspoon dried oregano
- Salt and pepper to taste
- Fresh basil leaves, for garnish (optional)

VARIATIONS

For added protein, top with grilled chicken or chickpeas. Substitute the tomato basil sauce with a pesto sauce for a different flavor profile. Add vegetables like spinach or mushrooms to the sauce for extra nutrition.

DIRECTIONS

1. Prepare Spaghetti Squash: Preheat the oven to 400°F (200°C). Cut the spaghetti squash in half lengthwise and remove the seeds. Drizzle with olive oil and season with salt and pepper. Place cut-side down on a baking sheet and roast for 40-45 minutes, or until tender.
2. Make Sauce: While the squash is roasting, heat olive oil in a skillet over medium heat. Add onion and cook until translucent, about 5 minutes. Add garlic and cook for another minute. Stir in diced tomatoes, tomato paste, dried basil, and oregano. Simmer for 15-20 minutes, allowing the flavors to meld. Season with salt and pepper to taste.
3. Combine: Once the squash is roasted, use a fork to scrape the flesh into spaghetti-like strands. Top with tomato basil sauce and garnish with fresh basil leaves if desired.

200 calories per serving, 5g protein, 10g fat, 25g carbohydrates, 6g fiber

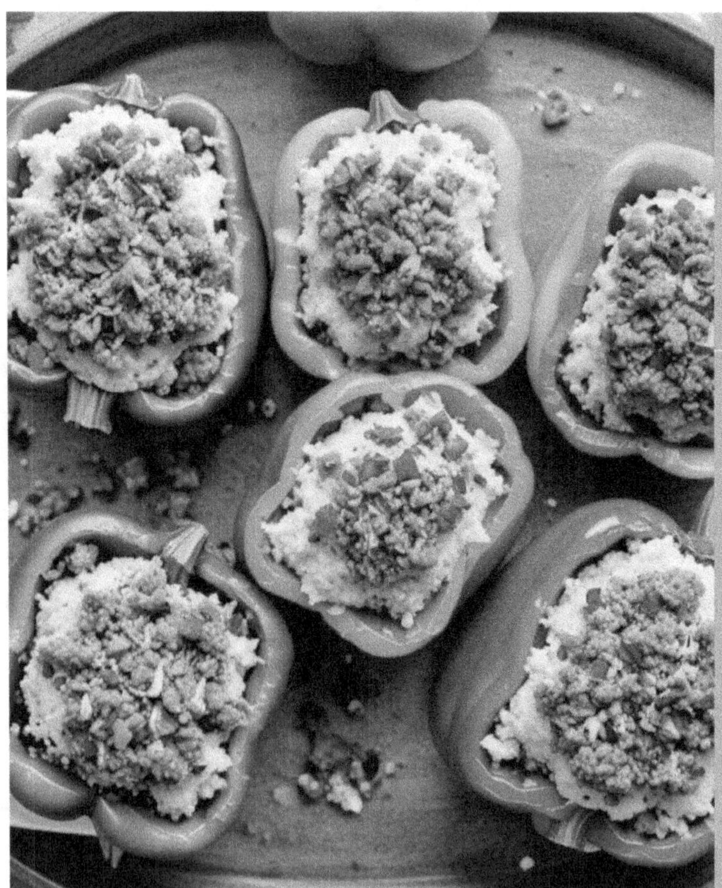

INGREDIENTS

- 4 large bell peppers (any color)
- 1 head cauliflower, riced (about 3 cups)
- 1 tablespoon olive oil
- 1 cup diced tomatoes
- 1 can (15 oz) black beans, drained and rinsed
- 1 cup corn kernels (fresh or frozen)
- 1 teaspoon ground cumin
- 1/2 teaspoon smoked paprika
- Salt and pepper to taste
- 1/2 cup shredded cheese (optional)
- Fresh cilantro, for garnish (optional)

VARIATIONS

Substitute cauliflower rice with quinoa or brown rice. Add other vegetables like mushrooms or zucchini to the stuffing mixture. For a spicier kick, add diced jalapeños or chili flakes.

DIRECTIONS

1. Prepare Peppers: Preheat the oven to 375°F (190°C). Cut the tops off the bell peppers and remove seeds and membranes. Set aside.
2. Prepare Cauliflower Rice: Heat olive oil in a skillet over medium heat. Add riced cauliflower and cook for 5-7 minutes, or until tender. Stir in diced tomatoes, black beans, corn, cumin, smoked paprika, salt, and pepper. Cook for an additional 5 minutes, allowing the flavors to combine.
3. Stuff Peppers: Spoon the cauliflower rice mixture into each bell pepper. Place the stuffed peppers in a baking dish. If using, sprinkle shredded cheese on top. Bake for 25-30 minutes, or until the peppers are tender and the cheese is melted.
4. Garnish: Garnish with fresh cilantro if desired before serving.

250 calories per serving, 10g protein, 7g fat, 35g carbohydrates, 9g fiber

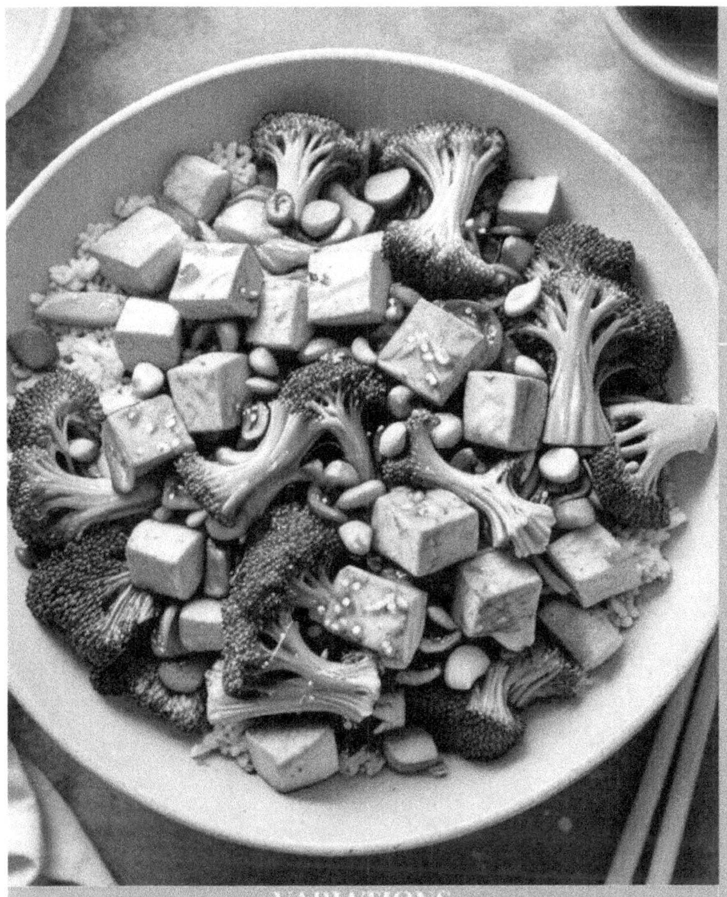

★★★★☆

Tofu Stir-Fry with Broccoli and Cashews

Prep Time	Cook Time

15 minutes	15 minutes

INGREDIENTS

- 1 block (14 oz) firm tofu, drained and cubed
- 2 tablespoons soy sauce or tamari
- 1 tablespoon olive oil
- 2 cups broccoli florets
- 1 red bell pepper, sliced
- 1 cup snap peas
- 1/2 cup cashews
- 2 tablespoons hoisin sauce
- 1 tablespoon rice vinegar
- 1 teaspoon grated ginger
- 2 cloves garlic, minced
- Cooked brown rice or quinoa, for serving

VARIATIONS

Substitute tofu with tempeh or chicken for a different protein source.
Add additional vegetables like carrots or mushrooms for variety.
Adjust the level of spice by adding chili paste or red pepper flakes.

DIRECTIONS

1. Marinate Tofu: In a bowl, toss tofu cubes with soy sauce or tamari. Let marinate for at least 10 minutes.
2. Cook Tofu: Heat olive oil in a large skillet or wok over medium-high heat. Add marinated tofu and cook for 5-7 minutes, or until golden brown on all sides. Remove tofu from the skillet and set aside.
3. Stir-Fry Vegetables: In the same skillet, add broccoli, red bell pepper, and snap peas. Stir-fry for 5-7 minutes, or until vegetables are crisp-tender.
4. Combine and Serve: Add tofu back to the skillet along with cashews, hoisin sauce, rice vinegar, ginger, and garlic. Stir well and cook for an additional 2-3 minutes, until heated through. Serve over brown rice or quinoa.

400 calories per serving, 20g protein, 20g fat, 35g carbohydrates, 5g fiber

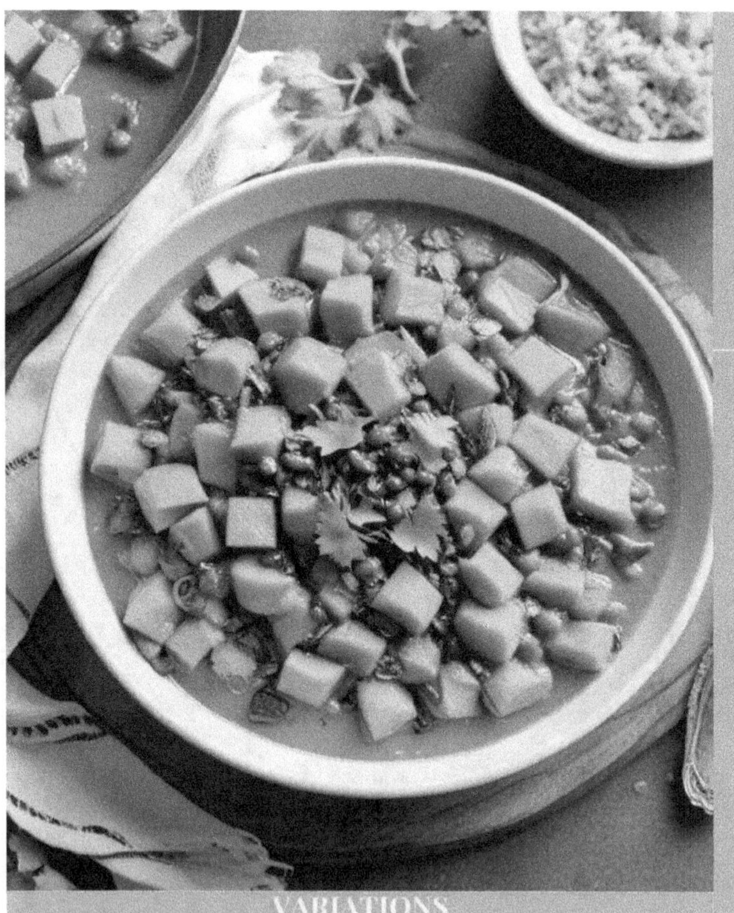

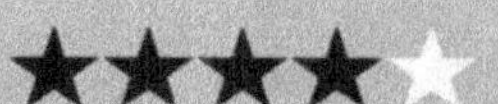

★★★★☆

Sweet and Spicy Butternut Squash Curry

Prep Time	Cook Time

15 minutes	30 minutes

INGREDIENTS

- 1 medium butternut squash, peeled and cubed
- 1 tablespoon coconut oil
- 1 onion, chopped
- 3 cloves garlic, minced
- 1 tablespoon ginger, minced
- 2 tablespoons curry powder
- 1 teaspoon ground cinnamon
- 1/2 teaspoon cayenne pepper (optional)
- 1 can (14 oz) coconut milk
- 1 can (14 oz) diced tomatoes
- 1 tablespoon maple syrup or honey
- Salt to taste
- Fresh cilantro, for garnish (optional)

VARIATIONS

For a heartier dish, add chickpeas or tofu. Adjust the sweetness and spice levels by modifying the amount of maple syrup and cayenne pepper. Serve with a side of rice or naan for a complete meal.

DIRECTIONS

1. Prepare Butternut Squash: In a large pot, heat coconut oil over medium heat. Add butternut squash cubes and cook for 5 minutes, stirring occasionally.
2. Sauté Aromatics: Add chopped onion, garlic, and ginger to the pot. Cook for 5 minutes, or until the onion is translucent.
3. Add Spices and Liquids: Stir in curry powder, cinnamon, and cayenne pepper. Cook for 1 minute to release the spices' aromas. Pour in coconut milk, diced tomatoes, and maple syrup. Bring to a boil, then reduce heat and simmer for 20-25 minutes, or until butternut squash is tender.
4. Season and Serve: Season with salt to taste. Garnish with fresh cilantro before serving.

300 calories per serving, 5g protein, 20g fat, 35g carbohydrates, 7g fiber

CHAPTER 5

Power-Packed Snacks

Roasted chickpeas with a spicy kick are a great option for a snack that's high in nutrients and taste. Garbanzo beans, also referred to as chickpeas, are a great source of fiber and plant-based protein. While fiber helps maintain a healthy weight, regulates blood sugar levels, and promotes digestive health, protein is essential for sustaining muscle mass and general physical functioning. Chickpeas are a great snack since roasting them brings out their flavor and gives them a nice crunch. Roasting chickpeas, as opposed to boiling or steaming, caramelizes their natural sugars, enhancing taste and increasing food enjoyment. , by removing moisture from the beans, the method gives them a crispy texture that fulfills the demands for crunchy snacks.

Another nutritious and convenient snack choice that is packed with power is an almond and date energy ball. Almonds are a great source of protein, healthy fats, and important elements including magnesium and vitamin E. These nutrients aid in muscular function, preserve energy levels and promote heart health. In addition to being naturally sweet and offering a rapid energy boost, dates also include dietary fiber, which promotes healthy digestion and helps keep blood sugar levels steady. These energy balls are a healthy snack because they include dates and almonds, which help to prevent the sugar surges that come with eating a lot of processed food. The extra benefits of making your energy balls are that they may be customized and don't include added sugar or preservatives, which are common in store-bought varieties. They are a flexible and healthy snack option since they can be produced with different ingredients to fit individual dietary requirements and taste preferences.

Hummus-topped veggie sticks provide a wholesome and filling snack that combines fresh veggies with a delicious dip. Carrots, celery, and bell peppers are examples of raw veggies that are high in vitamins, minerals, and fiber, all of which promote general health and well-being. To balance the crunchiness of the veggies, hummus, which is prepared with chickpeas, tahini, olive oil, lemon juice, and garlic, offers a rich taste and creamy texture. Protein and fiber are provided by the chickpeas in hummus, while other minerals like calcium and iron are provided by the tahini. This combo increases the snack's nutritious content and encourages fullness. To enhance the anti-cancer potential of hummus, contemplate blending in components such as flaxseeds or turmeric, which include anti-inflammatory and antioxidant characteristics. This change may increase the hummus's overall health benefits, making it a more potent snack in addition to being delicious.

A tasty and nutritious substitute for regular potato chips or other fried treats is baked kale chips. The leafy green vegetable kale is very nutrient-dense, offering a wealth of antioxidants, fiber, and vitamins A, C, and K. These nutrients help with digestion, strengthen the immune system, and promote good skin health, all of which are indicators of general health. When kale is baked instead of fried, it becomes crispy without using too much oil, which makes it a healthier option. Baking kale chips is a better way to retain the nutrients than frying, which may cause vitamins and other healthy ingredients to break down. Furthermore, baking enables the kale chips to be seasoned to personal preferences—from savory to spicy—without adding extra calories or bad fats.

These nutrient-dense, flavor-packed power snacks may promote a healthy lifestyle and help prevent cancer because of their wide range of nutritional advantages. By including these snacks in your diet, you may indulge in delicious delights while still enjoying satiating and healthful selections that support your objectives. All of the snacks are designed to provide vital nutrients and promote general health, so they're great options for anybody trying to add healthy, anti-cancer foods to their diet.

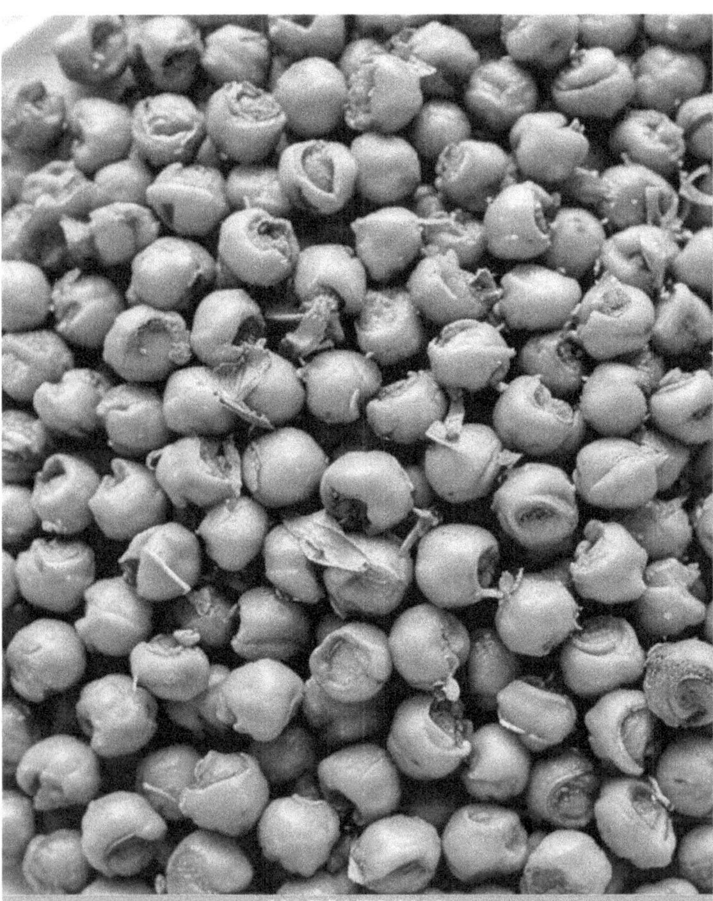

★★★★☆

Spicy Roasted Chickpeas

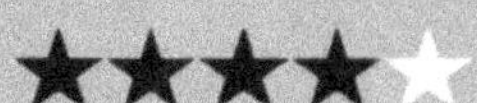

Prep Time
10 minutes

Cook Time
30 minutes

INGREDIENTS

- **1 can (15 oz) chickpeas, drained and rinsed**
- **2 tablespoons olive oil**
- **1 teaspoon smoked paprika**
- **1/2 teaspoon ground cumin**
- **1/2 teaspoon garlic powder**
- **1/4 teaspoon cayenne pepper (optional, for extra heat)**
- **Salt to taste**

VARIATIONS
Experiment with different spices like curry powder or chili lime seasoning for varied flavors. Add a touch of honey or maple syrup for a sweet-spicy blend.

DIRECTIONS

1. Preheat Oven: Preheat your oven to 400°F (200°C).
2. Prepare Chickpeas: Pat the chickpeas dry with a paper towel to remove excess moisture. This step is crucial for achieving a crispy texture.
3. Season: Toss the chickpeas with olive oil, smoked paprika, cumin, garlic powder, cayenne pepper (if using), and salt until evenly coated.
4. Roast: Spread the seasoned chickpeas in a single layer on a baking sheet. Roast for 25-30 minutes, shaking the pan halfway through to ensure even cooking.
5. Cool and Serve: Allow the chickpeas to cool slightly before enjoying them as a crunchy, protein-packed snack.

150 calories per serving (1/2 cup), 6g protein, 7g fat, 18g carbohydrates, 5g fiber

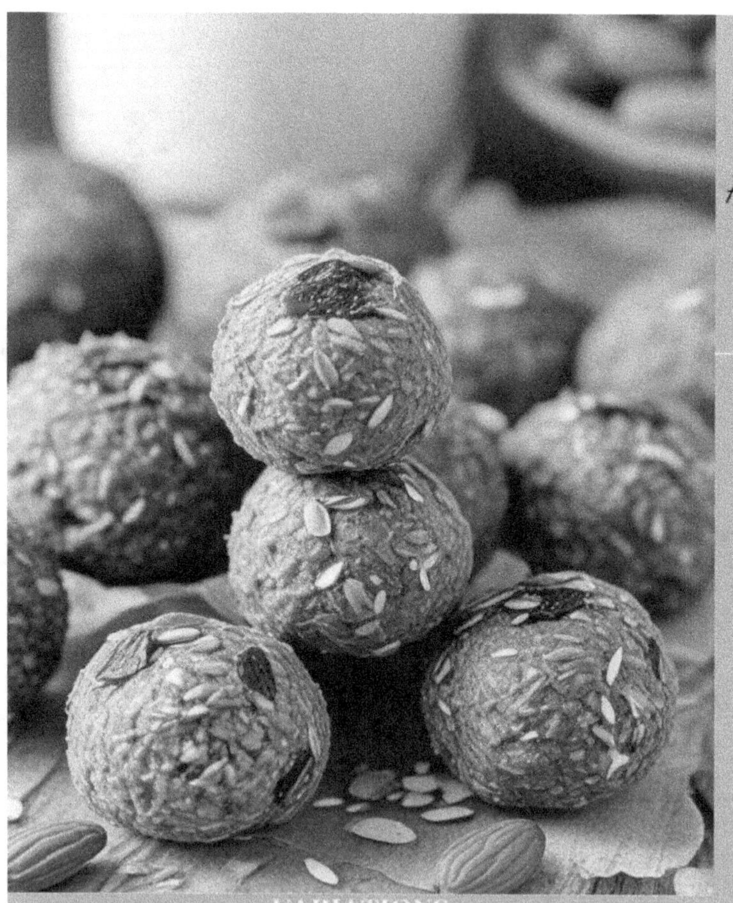

Almond and Date Energy Balls

Prep Time	Cook Time
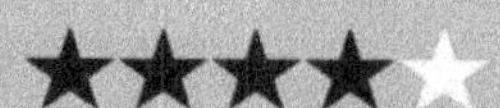 15 minutes	0 minutes

INGREDIENTS

- 1 cup almonds
- 1 cup pitted dates
- 1/4 cup unsweetened shredded coconut (optional)
- 1 tablespoon chia seeds (optional)
- 1/2 teaspoon vanilla extract

VARIATIONS

Substitute almonds with other nuts like cashews or walnuts. Add cacao powder for a chocolatey twist or mix in dried fruit like cranberries for added texture.

DIRECTIONS

1. Prepare Ingredients: Place almonds in a food processor and pulse until finely chopped. Add pitted dates and pulse until the mixture starts to stick together.
2. Blend: Add vanilla extract, and if using, shredded coconut and chia seeds. Process until the mixture is well combined and holds together when pressed.
3. Form Balls: Roll the mixture into 1-inch balls and place them on a parchment-lined baking sheet.
4. Chill: Refrigerate the energy balls for at least 30 minutes to firm up before serving.

100 calories per ball, 2g protein, 6g fat, 10g carbohydrates, 2g fiber

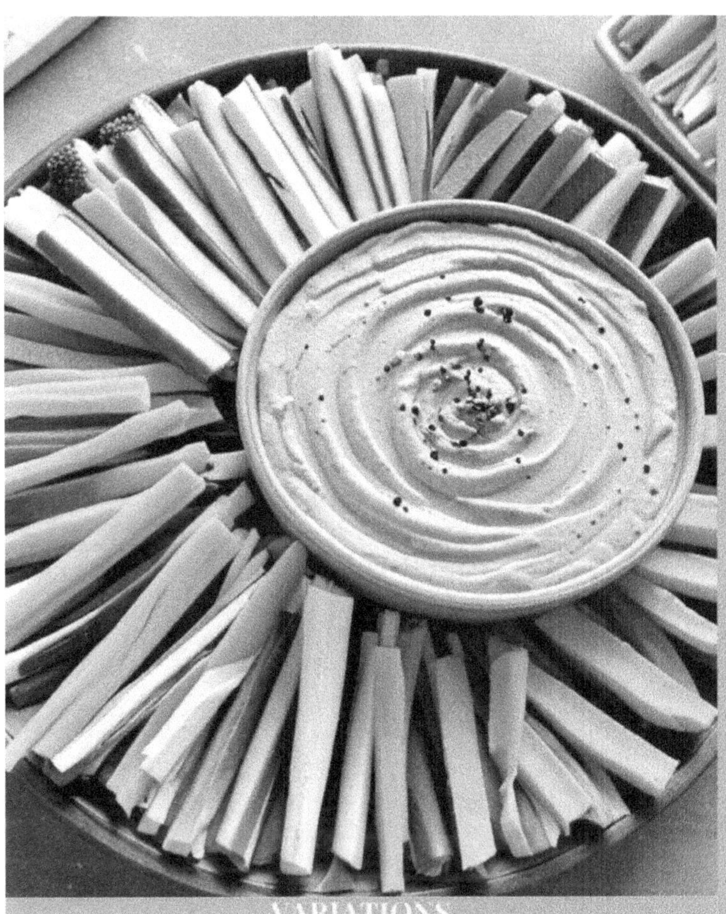

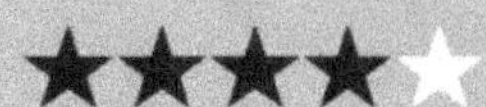

Veggie Sticks with Hummus

Prep Time
10 minutes

Cook Time
0 minutes

INGREDIENTS

- 1 cup baby carrots
- 1 cup celery sticks
- 1 cup bell pepper strips
- 1 cup cucumber sticks
- 1 cup homemade or store-bought hummus (see below for a simple recipe)

HUMMUS RECIPE (OPTIONAL)

- 1 can (15 oz) chickpeas, drained and rinsed
- 1/4 cup tahini
- 2 tablespoons olive oil
- 2 tablespoons lemon juice
- 2 cloves garlic, minced
- Salt to taste

DIRECTIONS

1. Prepare Vegetables: Wash and cut the vegetables into sticks or bite-sized pieces.
2. Serve: Arrange the veggie sticks on a plate or platter with a bowl of hummus for dipping.

INSTRUCTIONS FOR HUMMUS

1. Blend Ingredients: Combine all ingredients in a food processor and blend until smooth. Adjust seasoning and lemon juice as needed.
2. Serve: Transfer hummus to a bowl and serve with veggie sticks.

100 CALORIES PER SERVING (1/2 CUP HUMMUS WITH VEGGIE STICKS), 4G PROTEIN, 6G FAT, 12G CARBOHYDRATES, 4G FIBER

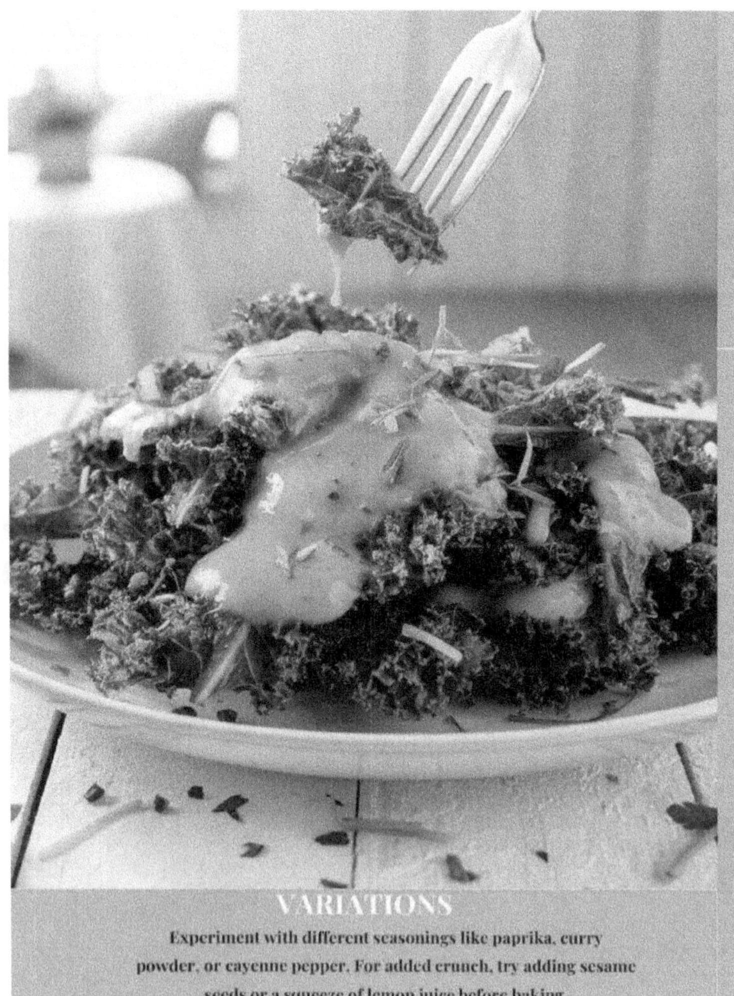

★★★★☆

Baked Kale Chips

Prep Time
10 minutes

Cook Time
15 minutes

INGREDIENTS

- 1 large bunch kale, stems removed and leaves torn into bite-sized pieces
- 1 tablespoon olive oil
- 1/2 teaspoon sea salt
- 1/4 teaspoon garlic powder (optional)
- 1/4 teaspoon nutritional yeast (optional, for a cheesy flavor)

VARIATIONS

Experiment with different seasonings like paprika, curry powder, or cayenne pepper. For added crunch, try adding sesame seeds or a squeeze of lemon juice before baking.

DIRECTIONS

1. Preheat Oven: Preheat your oven to 350°F (175°C).
2. Prepare Kale: Wash and thoroughly dry the kale leaves. Toss them with olive oil, salt, garlic powder, and nutritional yeast if using.
3. Bake: Spread the kale leaves in a single layer on a baking sheet. Bake for 10-15 minutes, or until crispy, turning once halfway through.
4. Cool and Enjoy: Allow kale chips to cool before eating. They will continue to crisp up as they cool.

100 calories per serving (1 cup), 4g protein, 7g fat, 8g carbohydrates, 3g fiber

CHAPTER 6

Satisfying Sides

Roasted herbs with garlic Brussels sprouts bring flavor and nutrients to any dish, making them a delicious addition. Brussels sprouts, a vegetable belonging to the cruciferous family, are high in fiber, antioxidants, and vitamins C and K. These nutrients are essential for maintaining the body's defenses against cancer, which come from nature. Brussels sprouts' high fiber content aids in digestive regulation and, by supporting a healthy gut microbiota, may help reduce the incidence of several cancers.

Brussels sprouts are a great side dish since roasting brings out their inherent sweetness and crisps them up. The taste profile is enhanced and the health benefits are multiplied when coupled with garlic and herbs. With its ability to reduce inflammation and increase antioxidant levels, garlic enhances the taste of Brussels sprouts and may help prevent cancer. Herbs like thyme and rosemary not only provide a taste explosion of freshness, but they also provide extra antioxidants that are good for your general health. This is a great way to prepare Brussels sprouts that enhances their flavor and improves their health.

Creamy avocado and cucumber soup is a nutrient-rich, pleasant side dish that has several health advantages. Monounsaturated fats, which are vital for heart health and maintaining a healthy weight, are abundant in avocados. These beneficial fats give the soup a creamy texture and aid in the absorption of fat-soluble vitamins. The abundant nutritional profile of avocados contains potassium, fiber, and vitamins E, C, and K, all of which support general health and may lower the risk of cancer.

When avocado and cucumber are combined in a soup, it produces a nutrient-dense, refreshing treat. In addition to adding a crisp taste, cucumbers are rich in water content, which aids in maintaining bodily hydration. It also offers a significant supply of minerals and vitamins, including potassium and vitamin K. This soup's perfect mix of good fats, water, and vital nutrients from the combination of avocado and cucumber makes it a filling and nutritious complement to any meal plan.

Carrots with a lemon-tahini glaze provide a special taste combination and health advantages. One of the most well-known benefits of carrots is their high beta-carotene concentration, which the body uses to make vitamin A. This vitamin is necessary to keep the immune system strong and to preserve good eyesight. Carrots also include antioxidants and fiber, which improve general health and may lower the risk of cancer.

Carrots are given a creamy texture and nutty taste with tahini, which is produced from sesame seeds. It has a lot of protein, good fats, and important minerals like iron and calcium. , chemicals in tahini have been shown to have antioxidant and anti-inflammatory qualities. Lemon juice not only adds brightness to the dish's taste but also provides vitamin C, which is essential for skin and immune system health. This meal is a tasty and nutritious side that benefits from the nutritional profile of the carrots provided by the addition of tahini and lemon.

A nutrient-dense side dish that goes well with a range of main dishes is quinoa and black bean salad. Quinoa is a beneficial complement to a plant-based diet since it is a complete protein source that contains all nine necessary amino acids. Moreover, it has significant quantities of antioxidants, fiber, and magnesium, all of which promote general health and help control blood sugar.

Another great source of fiber and protein is black beans. They are abundant in vitamins and minerals, including potassium, iron, and folate, which support a variety of body processes and help maintain a balanced diet. Quinoa and black beans combine to make a meal that is rich in fiber, which helps with digestion increases fullness, and is filled with protein. Because of its versatility, this salad may be made to suit diverse tastes by experimenting with different veggies and sauces.

There are several health advantages to including black bean salad with quinoa in a plant-based diet. It is a filling and nutritious choice since it offers a well-balanced blend of protein, fiber, and other nutrients. This salad is a great complement to any diet that focuses on cancer prevention and general well-being since it is not only tasty but also promotes overall health and well-being.

These side dishes, which include quinoa and black bean salad, lemon-tahini glazed carrots, creamy avocado, and cucumber soup, and roasted Brussels sprouts with garlic and herbs, each have their distinct tastes and nutritional advantages. A balanced and nutritious diet is enhanced by them since they provide vital nutrients that promote general health and perhaps lower the risk of cancer. These dishes are ideal for anybody wishing to add tasty and nutritious sides to their meals since they are meant to be both filling and nourishing.

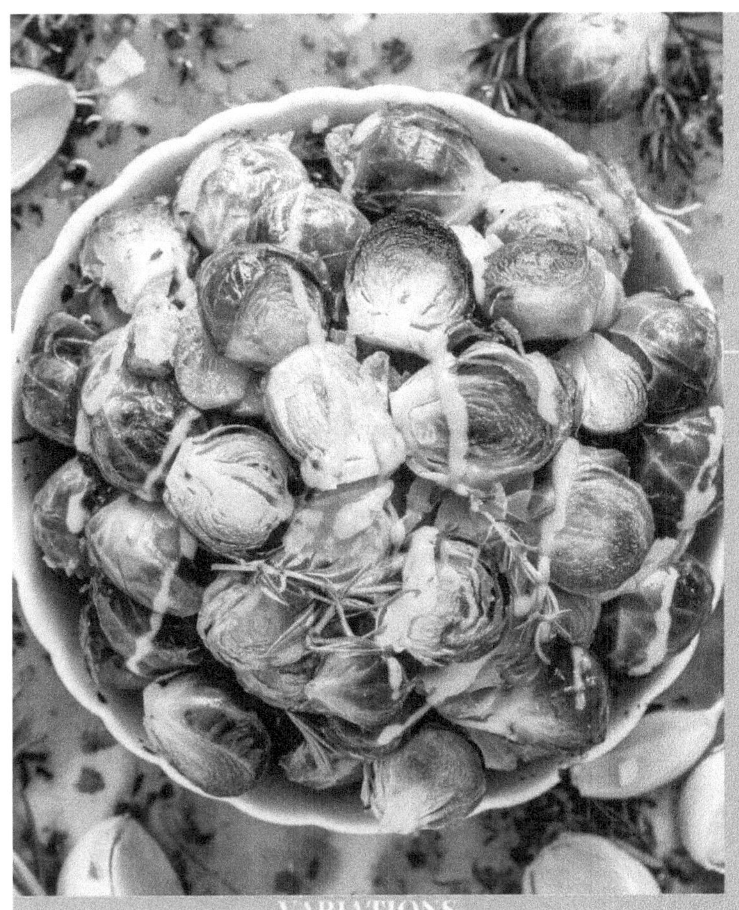

★★★★☆

Garlic and Herb Roasted
Brussels Sprouts

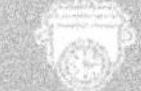

Prep Time	Cook Time
10 minutes	25 minutes

INGREDIENTS

- 1 lb Brussels sprouts, trimmed and halved
- 2 tablespoons olive oil
- 4 cloves garlic, minced
- 1 teaspoon dried rosemary
- 1 teaspoon dried thyme
- Salt and black pepper to taste

DIRECTIONS

1. Preheat Oven: Preheat your oven to 400°F (200°C).
2. Prepare Brussels Sprouts: Trim the Brussels sprouts by cutting off the ends and slicing them in half.
3. Season: In a large bowl, toss the Brussels sprouts with olive oil, minced garlic, rosemary, thyme, salt, and pepper until evenly coated.
4. Roast: Spread the seasoned Brussels sprouts on a baking sheet in a single layer. Roast in the preheated oven for 20-25 minutes, or until they are golden brown and crispy on the edges, shaking the pan halfway through.
5. Serve: Transfer to a serving dish and enjoy warm.

120 calories per serving (1 cup), 8g fat, 8g carbohydrates, 4g fiber, 4g protein

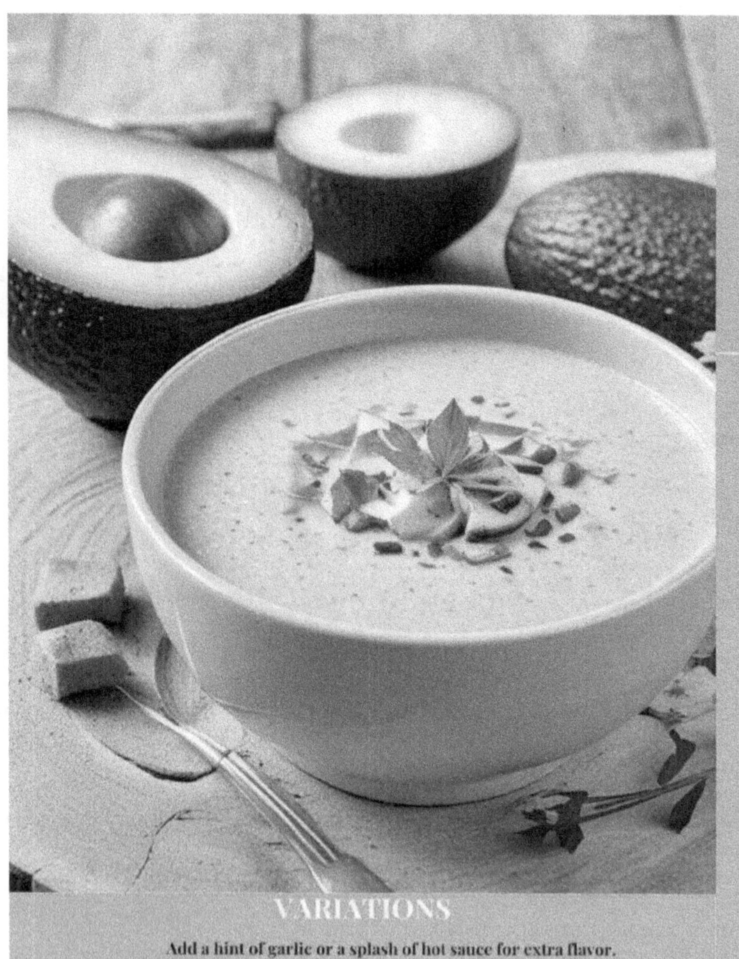

Creamy Avocado and Cucumber Soup

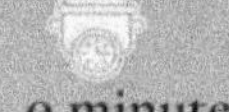

Prep Time	Cook Time
10 minutes	0 minutes

INGREDIENTS

- 2 ripe avocados, peeled and pitted
- 1 large cucumber, peeled and chopped
- 1 cup vegetable broth
- 1/4 cup fresh basil leaves
- 1 tablespoon lemon juice
- Salt and black pepper to taste

VARIATIONS

Add a hint of garlic or a splash of hot sauce for extra flavor. Incorporate other fresh herbs like cilantro or dill to change up the taste.

DIRECTIONS

1. Blend Ingredients: In a blender, combine the avocados, cucumber, vegetable broth, basil leaves, and lemon juice. Blend until smooth and creamy.
2. Season: Taste and adjust the seasoning with salt and pepper as needed.
3. Chill: For a colder soup, refrigerate for at least 30 minutes before serving.
4. Serve: Pour into bowls and garnish with additional basil leaves if desired.

200 calories per serving (1 cup), 14g fat, 15g carbohydrates, 7g fiber, 4g protein

Lemon-Tahini Glazed Carrots

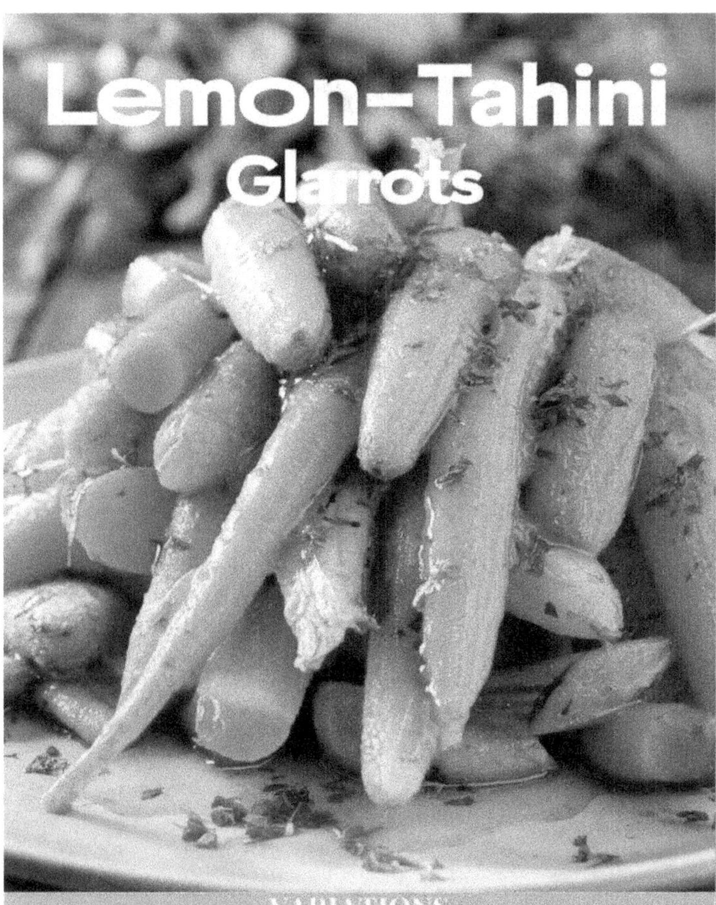

INGREDIENTS

- 1 lb carrots, peeled and sliced
- 2 tablespoons tahini
- 2 tablespoons lemon juice
- 1 tablespoon olive oil
- 1 tablespoon maple syrup (optional, for added sweetness)
- Salt and black pepper to taste

DIRECTIONS

1. Prepare Carrots: Preheat oven to 375°F (190°C). Toss the carrot slices with a little olive oil, salt, and pepper. Spread on a baking sheet.
2. Roast Carrots: Roast in the oven for 20–25 minutes, or until tender and slightly caramelized.
3. Prepare Glaze: In a small bowl, whisk together tahini, lemon juice, olive oil, and maple syrup if using.
4. Glaze Carrots: Once the carrots are roasted, drizzle the tahini glaze over them and toss to coat evenly.
5. Serve: Transfer to a serving dish and enjoy warm.

180 calories per serving (1 cup), 11g fat, 20g carbohydrates, 6g fiber, 3g protein

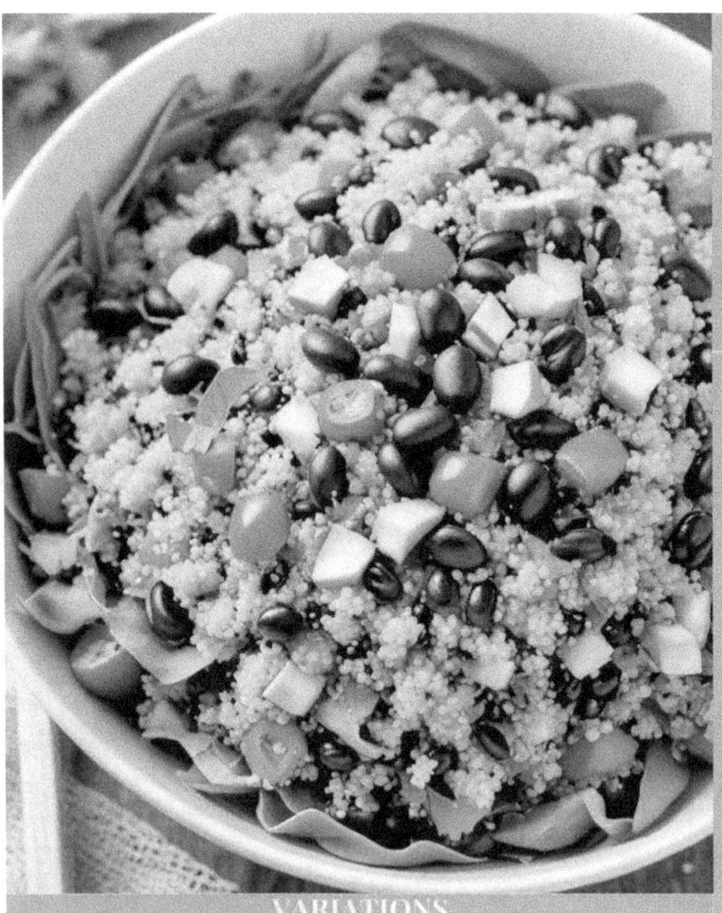

Quinoa and Black Bean Salad

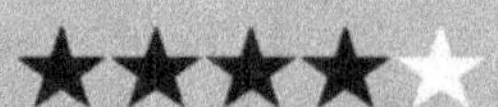

Prep Time	Cook Time
15 minutes	15 minutes

INGREDIENTS

- 1 cup quinoa
- 1 can (15 oz) black beans, drained and rinsed
- 1 cup corn kernels (fresh or frozen)
- 1 red bell pepper, diced
- 1/4 cup red onion, finely chopped
- 1/4 cup fresh cilantro, chopped
- Juice of 1 lime
- 2 tablespoons olive oil
- Salt and black pepper to taste

VARIATIONS

Add diced avocado for extra creaminess or mix in some chopped tomatoes for added freshness. For a spicier kick, include a diced jalapeño pepper or a pinch of chili powder.

DIRECTIONS

1. Cook Quinoa: Rinse quinoa under cold water. In a medium pot, bring 2 cups of water to a boil. Add quinoa, reduce heat, cover, and simmer for about 15 minutes, or until the water is absorbed and quinoa is tender. Fluff with a fork and let cool.
2. Combine Ingredients: In a large bowl, combine the cooled quinoa, black beans, corn, red bell pepper, red onion, and cilantro.
3. Dress Salad: In a small bowl, whisk together lime juice, olive oil, salt, and pepper. Pour over the salad and toss to combine.
4. Serve: Chill for at least 30 minutes before serving to allow flavors to meld.

220 calories per serving (1 cup). 7g fat, 30g carbohydrates, 8g fiber, 8g protein

CHAPTER 7

Delicious Desserts

Rich and creamy, dark chocolate avocado mousse is a decadent treat that also happens to be healthy. The key ingredient that gives this mousse its smooth, creamy texture without requiring a lot of heavy cream is avocado. Apart from improving texture, avocado has several other health advantages. Full of fiber, potassium, vitamin E, and other vital vitamins and minerals, it is also high in heart-healthy monounsaturated fats. These nutrients have been associated with decreased inflammation, heart health, and general well-being.

Antioxidant qualities of dark chocolate, especially those with a high cocoa content, are well known. Flavonoids are substances found in it that can counteract free radicals and lessen oxidative stress in the body. In addition to improving general health, this may reduce the chance of developing chronic illnesses, such as certain forms of cancer. Not only does avocado and dark chocolate combine to form a deliciously rich and creamy dessert, but it also has many health advantages that make it a guilt-free indulgence.

Almond butter with berry chia jam is another treat that perfectly combines taste and health. The main component in this jam, chia seeds, is a nutritional powerhouse. They contain a lot of omega-3 fatty acids, which are well-known for their heart-healthy advantages and anti-inflammatory qualities. , chia seeds include a significant quantity of fiber, which aids with digestion and keeps blood sugar levels steady. They also support general health as a wonderful source of vitamins, minerals, and antioxidants.

The nutritional profile of the jam is improved when it is served with almond butter. Protein and good fats from almond butter assist in keeping you full and provide you with energy that lasts. In addition, it has magnesium, vitamin E, and other vital minerals that assist several body processes. This combination produces a dessert that is filling and healthy in addition to being a delightful spread.

A popular dish that puts a healthy spin on holiday favorites is apple cinnamon crumble. The primary component, apples, are a great source of vitamin C and nutritional fiber. , they include a variety of antioxidants that may help prevent cancer and promote heart health. Because apples are naturally sweet, less extra sugar is required, making this a healthier dessert choice.

An essential component of the crumble topping, cinnamon has several health advantages of its own. It has ingredients that have been shown to have antioxidant and anti-inflammatory qualities. Research indicates that cinnamon may have a positive impact on insulin sensitivity and blood sugar regulation, which may help manage and prevent diabetes. Its fragrant, warming properties also provide a lovely taste that harmonizes well with the apples.

A cool and delightful treat that transports you to a tropical paradise is coconut mango sorbet. Because of its high-fat content, coconut gives the sorbet a rich, creamy texture. Medium-chain triglycerides (MCTs), which are mostly found in coconut oil, are recognized for their potential advantages in promoting metabolic health and supplying rapid energy. In addition to adding a nice texture and a hint of sweetness, coconut makes the sorbet both decadent and healthful.

The major component in this delicacy, the mango, is loaded with vitamins A and C, which are essential for immune system health and beautiful skin. Antioxidants like beta-carotene, which promotes eye health and may aid in the prevention of certain cancers, are also abundant in mangos. This sorbet, which combines mango and coconut, is a wonderful and healthy dish that promotes overall health while allowing you to experience the natural sweetness of fruit.

These desserts, which include coconut mango sorbet, apple cinnamon crumble, berry chia jam with almond butter, and dark chocolate avocado mousse, each provide a distinctive opportunity to indulge in sweets while simultaneously gaining health advantages. These dishes are a great option for anybody who wants to enjoy them without sacrificing their nutritional objectives since they combine tasty tastes with components that promote wellbeing.

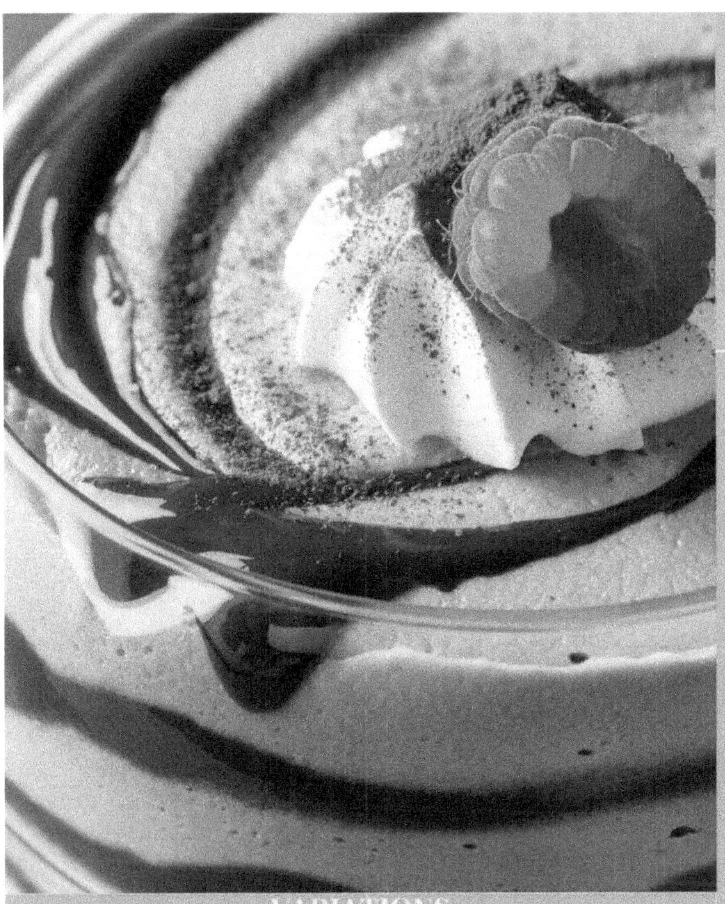

★★★★☆

Dark Chocolate Avocado Mousse

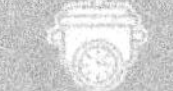

Prep Time

10 minutes

Cook Time

0 minutes

INGREDIENTS

- 2 ripe avocados
- 1/2 cup dark chocolate chips or chopped dark chocolate (70% cocoa or higher)
- 1/4 cup pure maple syrup or honey
- 1/4 cup unsweetened cocoa powder
- 1 teaspoon vanilla extract
- Pinch of salt

VARIATIONS

For a different flavor, try adding a pinch of espresso powder or a few tablespoons of almond butter to the mixture. For a lighter texture, fold in some whipped coconut cream before chilling.

DIRECTIONS

1. Melt Chocolate: In a microwave-safe bowl, melt the dark chocolate in 20-second intervals, stirring in between until smooth. Alternatively, melt the chocolate using a double boiler.
2. Blend Ingredients: Scoop the flesh from the avocados and place it in a blender or food processor. Add the melted chocolate, maple syrup or honey, cocoa powder, vanilla extract, and a pinch of salt.
3. Process: Blend until the mixture is completely smooth and creamy. Taste and adjust sweetness or cocoa powder if needed.
4. Chill: Spoon the mousse into serving dishes and refrigerate for at least 30 minutes to allow it to set.
5. Serve: Garnish with fresh berries, mint leaves, or a sprinkle of sea salt if desired.

250 calories per serving (1/2 cup), 20g fat, 20g carbohydrates, 8g fiber, 3g protein

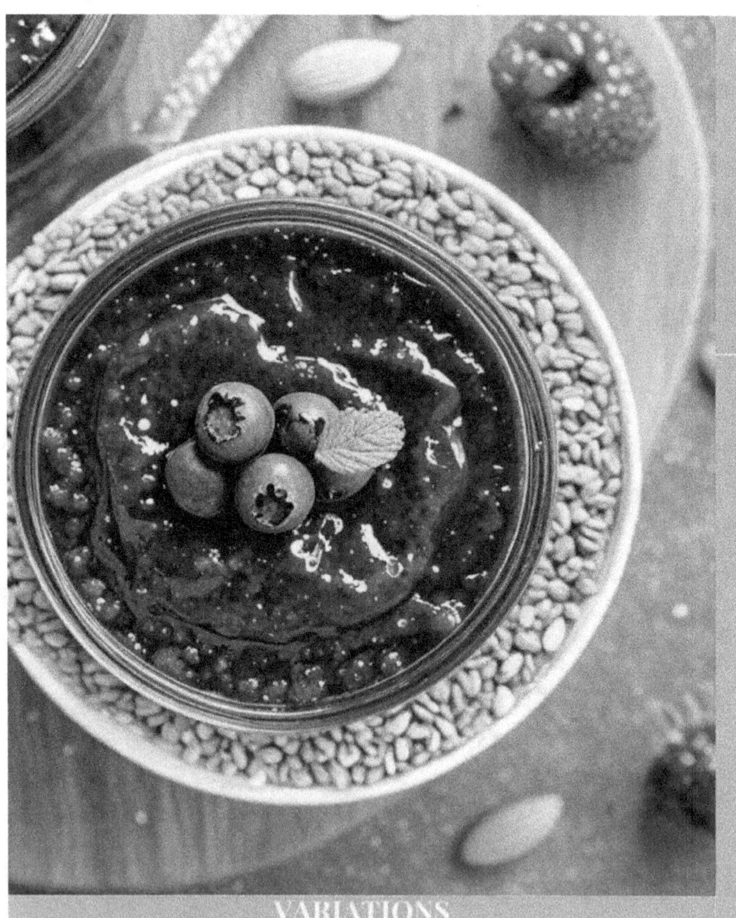

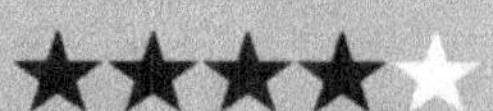

★★★★☆

Berry Chia Jam with Almond Butter

Prep Time

10 minutes

Cook Time

15 minutes

INGREDIENTS

- 2 cups mixed berries (fresh or frozen)
- 1/4 cup chia seeds
- 2 tablespoons maple syrup or honey
- 1 teaspoon lemon juice
- 1/4 cup almond butter

DIRECTIONS

1. Cook Berries: In a medium saucepan, combine the berries and maple syrup. Cook over medium heat until the berries break down and release their juices, about 5-7 minutes.
2. Add Chia Seeds: Stir in the chia seeds and lemon juice. Continue to cook for an additional 5 minutes, stirring occasionally, until the mixture thickens.
3. Cool and Blend: Remove from heat and let the mixture cool slightly. Blend with an immersion blender or regular blender until smooth, if desired.
4. Add Almond Butter: Stir in the almond butter until well combined.
5. Store: Transfer the jam to a jar and refrigerate. It will continue to thicken as it cools.

150 calories per serving (2 tablespoons), 8g fat, 20g carbohydrates, 6g fiber, 4g protein

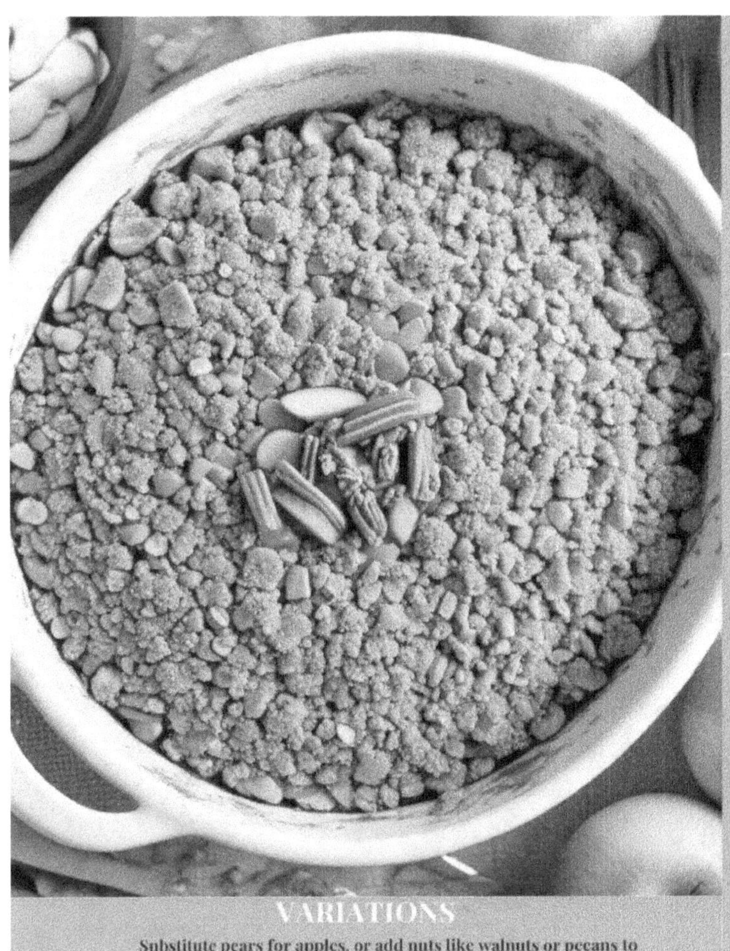

★★★★☆

Apple Cinnamon Crumble

Prep Time	Cook Time
15 minutes	40 minutes

INGREDIENTS

For the Filling:

- 4 large apples, peeled, cored, and sliced
- 1 tablespoon lemon juice
- 1/4 cup maple syrup or honey
- 1 teaspoon ground cinnamon
- 1/4 teaspoon ground nutmeg

For the Crumble Topping:

- 1 cup rolled oats
- 1/2 cup almond flour
- 1/4 cup coconut oil or butter
- 1/4 cup maple syrup or honey
- 1/4 teaspoon salt

VARIATIONS

Substitute pears for apples, or add nuts like walnuts or pecans to the crumble topping for added crunch. For a sweeter topping, increase the amount of maple syrup or honey.

DIRECTIONS

1. Preheat Oven: Preheat your oven to 350°F (175°C).
2. Prepare Filling: In a large bowl, toss the sliced apples with lemon juice, maple syrup, cinnamon, and nutmeg until well coated. Transfer to a baking dish.
3. Make Topping: In a separate bowl, combine the oats, almond flour, coconut oil, maple syrup, and salt. Mix until the mixture resembles coarse crumbs.
4. Assemble: Sprinkle the crumble topping evenly over the apple mixture.
5. Bake: Bake in the preheated oven for 35-40 minutes, or until the topping is golden brown and the apples are tender.
6. Serve: Allow to cool slightly before serving. Enjoy warm or at room temperature.

220 calories per serving (1/2 cup). 10g fat, 30g carbohydrates. 5g fiber, 2g protein

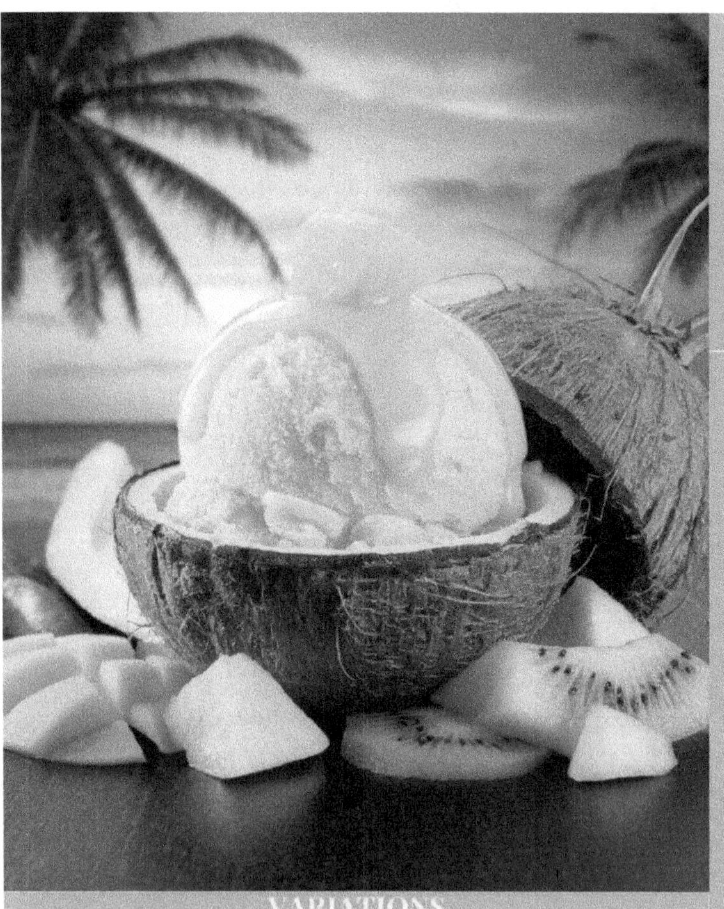

★★★★☆

Coconut Mango Sorbet

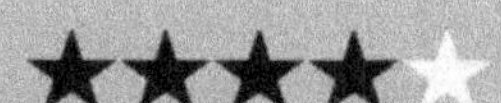

Prep Time
10 minutes

Cook Time
0 minutes

INGREDIENTS

- 2 ripe mangoes, peeled and chopped
- 1 cup coconut milk (canned or full-fat)
- 1/4 cup lime juice
- 1/4 cup honey or agave syrup
- 1 teaspoon vanilla extract

DIRECTIONS

1. Blend Ingredients: In a blender or food processor, combine the mangoes, coconut milk, lime juice, honey, and vanilla extract. Blend until smooth.
2. Freeze: Pour the mixture into a shallow dish or ice cream maker. If using a shallow dish, freeze for about 4 hours, stirring every 30 minutes to break up ice crystals. If using an ice cream maker, churn according to the manufacturer's instructions.
3. Serve: Once the sorbet has reached the desired consistency, scoop into bowls and enjoy.

150 calories per serving (1/2 cup), 9g fat, 19g carbohydrates, 2g fiber, 1g protein

CHAPTER 8

Beverages and Smoothies

A colorful concoction of nutrient-dense fruits and vegetables, detox green juice may help the body's natural detoxification processes and may even protect against cancer. Usually, kale, spinach, cucumber, celery, green apple, and lemon are the main components. Antioxidants and phytochemicals included in kale and spinach help prevent oxidative stress, which is linked to the development of cancer. These leafy greens are rich in folate, fiber, and vitamins A, C, and K, all of which enhance immune system function and general cellular health.

Due to their high water content, celery and cucumber help the body eliminate toxins and improve hydration. The green apple contributes vitamin C, which is necessary for healthy skin and the immune system, as well as a hint of natural sweetness. Because lemon juice has a high concentration of vitamin C and citric acid, it helps with digestion and improves the absorption of vital nutrients, which further assists detoxification.

Including green juice in your daily routine will help you increase the amount of essential nutrients you consume and aid in the process of detoxifying. Because of the juice's concentrated mixture of fruits and vegetables, eating a lot of greens—which might be difficult to fit into your diet otherwise—is made simple. Green juice is a healthy complement to any lifestyle that emphasizes health since it may help support liver function, enhance digestion, and boost energy levels when used regularly.

The potent anti-inflammatory and immune-boosting characteristics of turmeric are combined with the calming effects of a latte to create a warm, pleasant immune-boosting turmeric latte. Curcumin, a substance with strong anti-inflammatory and antioxidant properties, is found in turmeric. It has been shown that curcumin inhibits the development of cancer cells and improves the body's defenses against inflammation and infections.

Turmeric is mixed with milk or a dairy-free substitute, such as almond or oat milk, plus spices like cinnamon and black pepper to make a latte. Piperine, found in black pepper, greatly increases the absorption of curcumin, increasing the potency of turmeric. While the milk or milk substitute lends a creamy texture and more nutrients, cinnamon offers more antioxidants and a delicious taste.

If you're not a big lover of turmeric's strong taste in other foods, the latte format provides a fun and easy way to include it in your diet. Having a turmeric latte may be a calming routine that improves digestion, boosts immunity generally, and may help with inflammation-related ailments. For individuals looking for a warm, nourishing beverage that supports their health objectives, it's a great choice.

A berry-beet smoothie is a nutrient-dense beverage that promotes both cancer prevention and general wellness by combining the antioxidant-rich properties of berries with the detoxifying properties of beets. Strawberries, raspberries, and blueberries are just a few of the berries that are abundant in vitamins, minerals, and antioxidants called anthocyanins. These compounds have been connected to a lower risk of cancer and better heart health. They also include fiber, which promotes healthy digestion and steady blood sugar levels.

The high concentration of betalains, on the other hand, is well recognized to promote liver function and aid in the body's detoxification process. Nitrates, which may enhance blood flow and reduce blood pressure, are also included in them. Berries and beets together provide a tasty and nutritious smoothie that is packed with minerals like potassium, vitamin C, and folate.

Increasing antioxidant consumption, enhancing digestion, and promoting cardiovascular health, including a berry beet smoothie in your regular diet may improve your general health. A healthy complement to any routine, the smoothie is a pleasant and adaptable choice that may be consumed as a nutritional snack or as a meal substitute.

Cucumber's hydration qualities and mint's calming taste combine to create a delightful and easy drink called hydrating cucumber mint water. Since water makes up the majority of cucumber, it's a great food to eat to remain hydrated. , it has anti-inflammatory and antioxidant properties that promote skin health and cleansing.

In addition to adding taste, mint has been used historically to ease stomach pain and promote better digestion. It also imparts a subtle sweetness without the need for extra sugar. Cucumber and mint infusions make water taste good and promote drinking more water, which is important for being well-hydrated and for good health in general.

Cucumber mint water has advantages that go beyond simple hydration. Frequent use may aid in cleaning the skin, maintain a healthy digestive system, and provide a pleasant substitute for sugar-filled drinks. It's a fun and simple way to remain hydrated and enjoy the health advantages of natural ingredients.

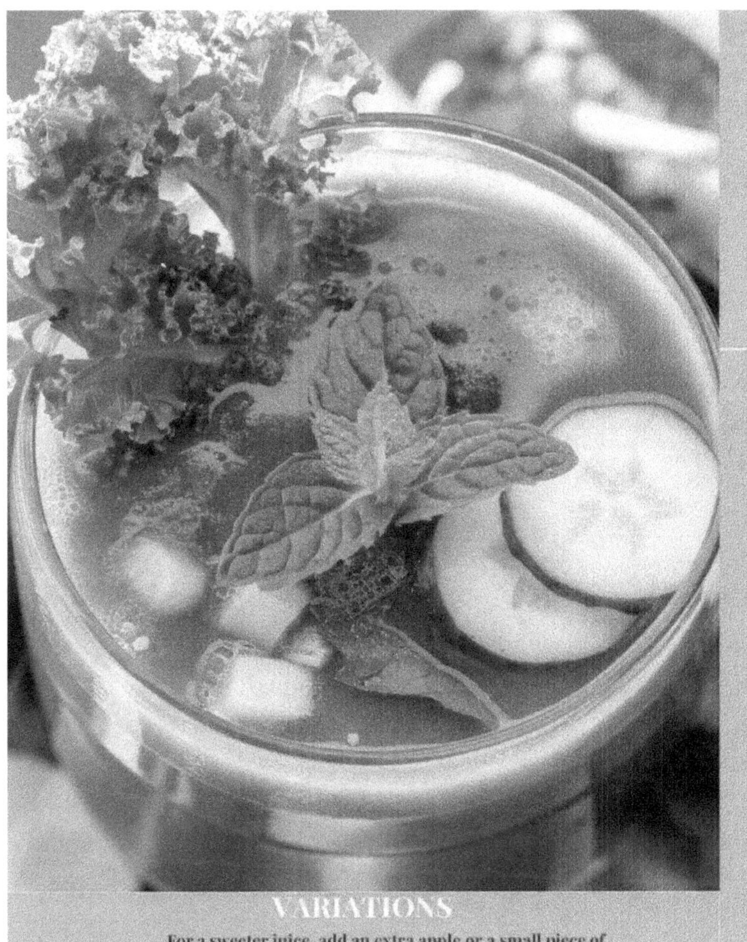

DIRECTIONS

1. Prepare Ingredients: Wash and chop all the vegetables and fruits.
2. Juice: In a juicer, combine the kale, spinach, cucumber, celery, green apple, and ginger. Juice until smooth.
3. Add Lemon: Stir in the lemon juice.
4. Mix with Water: Dilute with water or coconut water if needed to achieve desired consistency.
5. Serve: Pour into glasses and enjoy immediately for the freshest taste and maximum nutrient benefits.

80 calories per serving (1 cup), 0.5g fat, 20g carbohydrates, 4g fiber, 3g protein

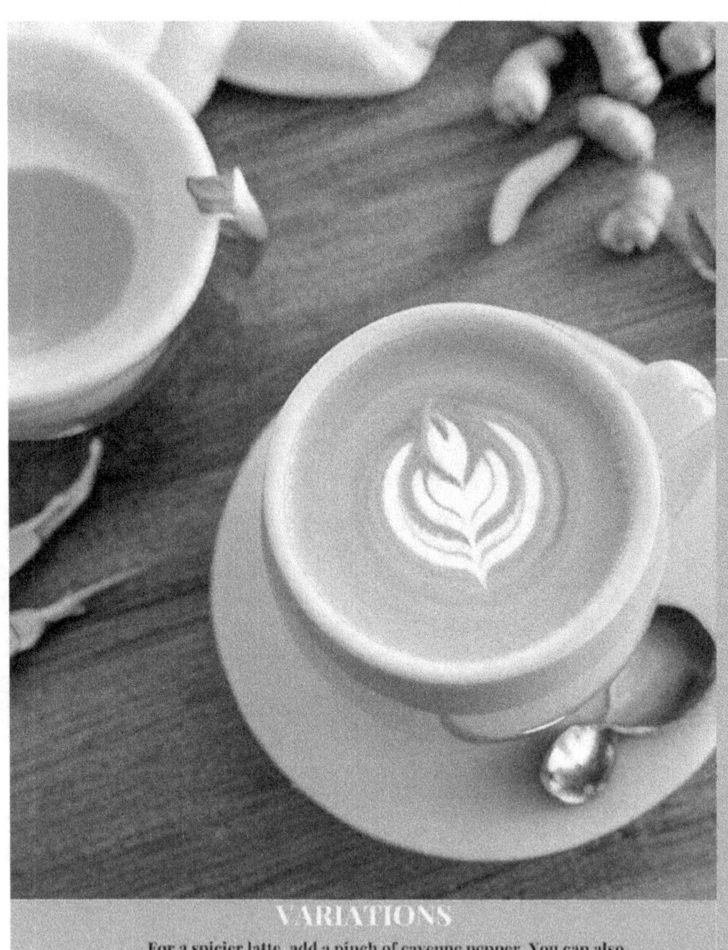

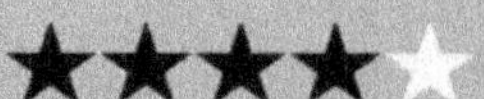

★★★★☆

Immune-Boosting Turmeric Latte

Prep Time

5 minutes

Cook Time

5 minutes

INGREDIENTS

- 1 cup almond milk (or other plant-based milk)
- 1 teaspoon ground turmeric
- 1/2 teaspoon ground cinnamon
- 1/4 teaspoon black pepper
- 1 tablespoon honey or maple syrup
- 1/2 teaspoon vanilla extract

VARIATIONS

For a spicier latte, add a pinch of cayenne pepper. You can also use coconut milk for a creamier texture or blend the latte for a frothy finish.

DIRECTIONS

1. Heat Milk: In a small saucepan, heat the almond milk over medium heat until hot but not boiling.
2. Mix Spices: In a small bowl, whisk together the turmeric, cinnamon, and black pepper.
3. Combine: Add the spice mixture to the hot almond milk, stirring well to combine.
4. Sweeten: Stir in the honey or maple syrup and vanilla extract.
5. Serve: Pour into a mug and enjoy warm.

100 calories per serving, 3g fat, 18g carbohydrates, 0g fiber, 1g protein

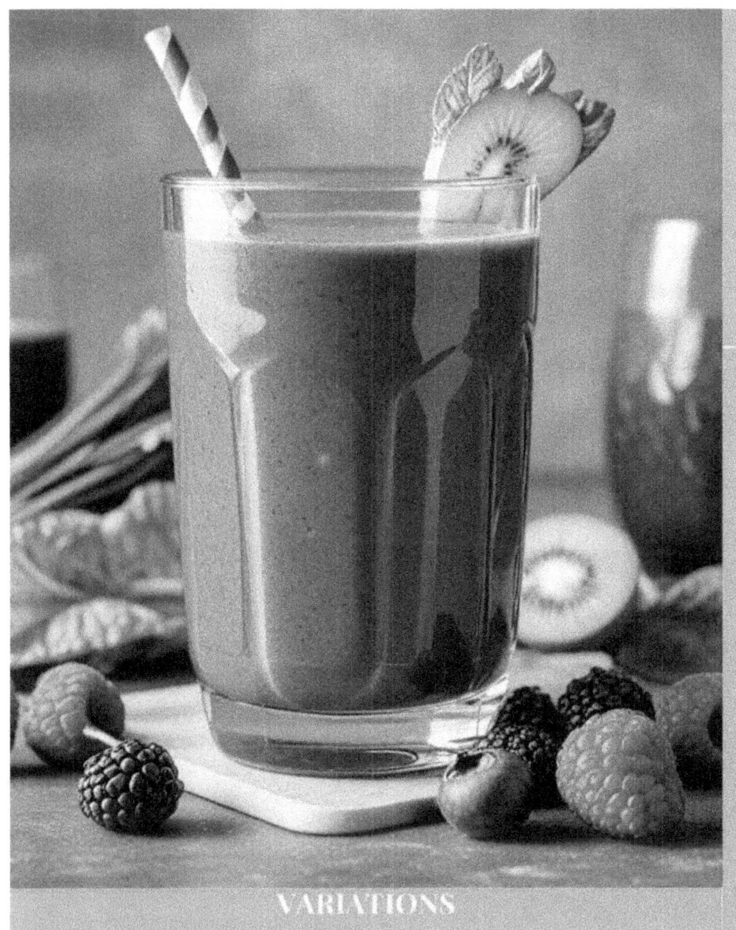

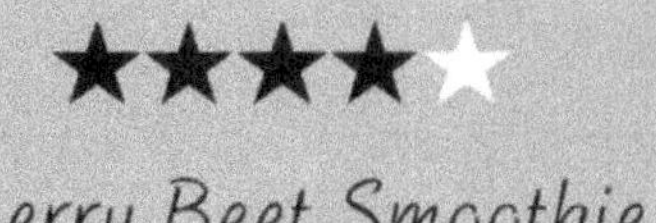

★★★★☆

Berry Beet Smoothie

Prep Time
10 minutes

Cook Time
10 minutes

INGREDIENTS

- 1 cup mixed berries (fresh or frozen)
- 1 small beet, peeled and chopped
- 1 banana
- 1/2 cup Greek yogurt or a dairy-free alternative
- 1 tablespoon chia seeds
- 1 cup almond milk or water
- 1 tablespoon honey or agave syrup (optional)

DIRECTIONS

1. Prepare Beet: Steam or boil the beet until tender. Let it cool slightly.
2. Blend Ingredients: In a blender, combine the berries, beet, banana, Greek yogurt, chia seeds, and almond milk.
3. Sweeten: Add honey or agave syrup if additional sweetness is desired.
4. Blend: Blend until smooth and creamy.
5. Serve: Pour into glasses and enjoy immediately.

250 calories per serving (1 cup), 5g fat, 40g carbohydrates, 8g fiber, 8g protein

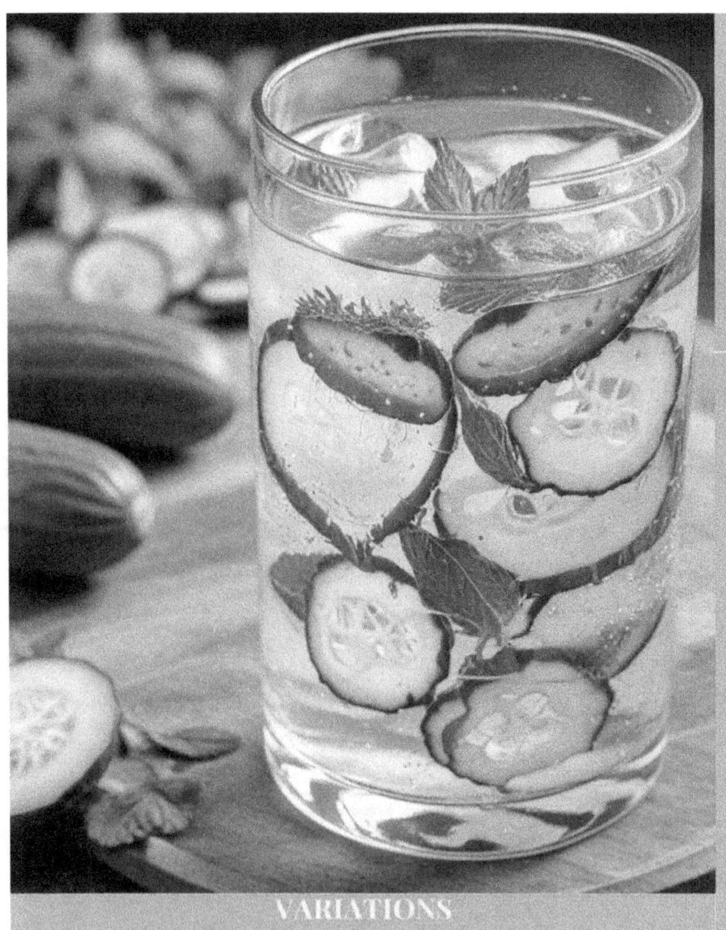

DIRECTIONS

1. Prepare Ingredients: Slice the cucumber and lemon, and gently bruise the mint leaves to release their flavor.
2. Combine: In a large pitcher, combine the cucumber slices, mint leaves, and lemon slices.
3. Add Water: Pour in the water and stir gently.
4. Infuse: Refrigerate for at least 2 hours to allow the flavors to meld.
5. Serve: Pour into glasses with ice if desired.

0 calories per serving (1 cup), 0g fat, 0g carbohydrates, 0g fiber, 0g protein

CHAPTER 9

Low Glycemic Recipes

Foods low in glycemic index are essential for controlling blood sugar levels, which is advantageous for those who are trying to avoid or treat cancer. These meals assist in preserving stable blood glucose levels and lower the chance of inflammation, which is connected to the advancement of cancer. Including low-glycemic items in your diet may also help you maintain a healthy weight, enhance insulin sensitivity, and promote overall metabolic health.

Replace high-glycemic items with slower-digesting alternatives to modify recipes and reduce their glycemic index. Choose whole grains over processed grains, utilize high-fiber vegetables and legumes to balance your consumption of carbohydrates, and swap out sugary ingredients with low-glycemic sweeteners like stevia or monk fruit.

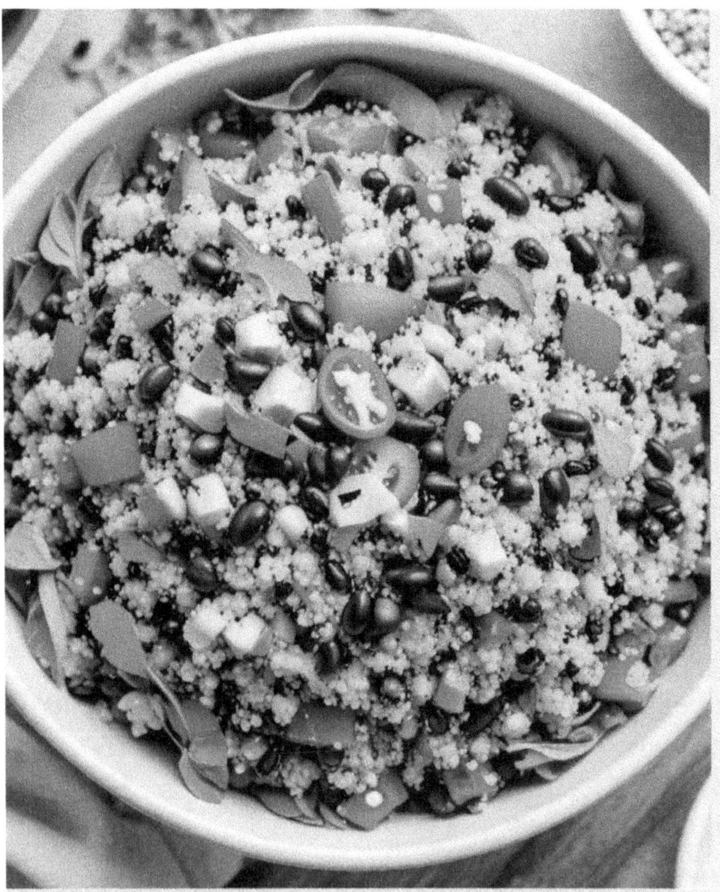

★★★★☆

Prep Time

15 minutes

Cook Time

15 minutes

INGREDIENTS

- 1 cup quinoa
- 1 can (15 oz) black beans, drained and rinsed
- 1 red bell pepper, diced
- 1/2 cup chopped fresh cilantro
- 1/4 cup lime juice
- 2 tablespoons olive oil
- 1 teaspoon cumin
- Salt and pepper to taste

NUTRITIONAL INFORMATION
280 CALORIES PER SERVING (1 CUP), 8G FAT, 35G
CARBOHYDRATES, 8G FIBER, 12G PROTEIN

DIRECTIONS

1. Cook Quinoa: Rinse quinoa under cold water. In a medium saucepan, combine quinoa with 2 cups of water. Bring to a boil, reduce heat, cover, and simmer for 15 minutes. Let it cool.
2. Mix Ingredients: In a large bowl, combine the cooked quinoa, black beans, red bell pepper, and cilantro.
3. Prepare Dressing: In a small bowl, whisk together lime juice, olive oil, cumin, salt, and pepper.
4. Combine and Serve: Pour the dressing over the salad and toss to combine. Serve chilled or at room temperature.

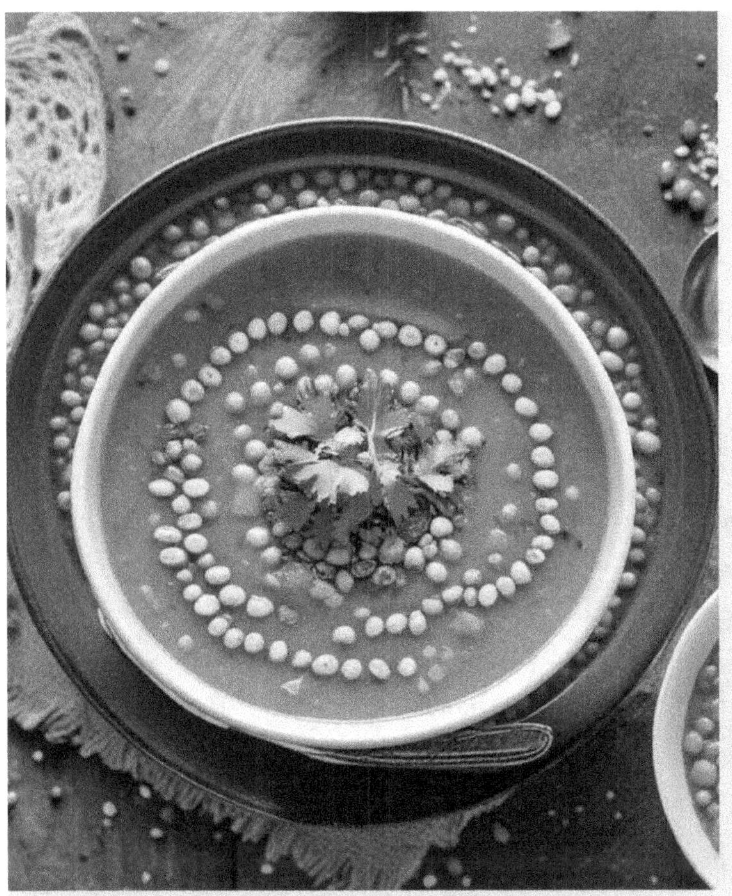

★★★★

Spicy Lentil Soup

Prep Time	Cook Time
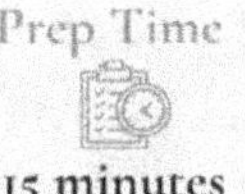	
15 minutes	30 minutes

INGREDIENTS

- 1 cup dried green or brown lentils
- 1 tablespoon olive oil
- 1 onion, chopped
- 2 cloves garlic, minced
- 1 carrot, diced
- 1 celery stalk, diced
- 1 can (14.5 oz) diced tomatoes
- 4 cups vegetable broth
- 1 teaspoon paprika
- 1/2 teaspoon cayenne pepper (optional)
- Salt and pepper to taste

DIRECTIONS

1. Cook Lentils: Rinse lentils and set aside.
2. Sauté Vegetables: In a large pot, heat olive oil over medium heat. Add onion and garlic, cooking until softened.
3. Add Veggies: Stir in carrot and celery, cooking for another 5 minutes.
4. Simmer Soup: Add diced tomatoes, vegetable broth, lentils, paprika, and cayenne pepper. Bring to a boil, then reduce heat and simmer for 25-30 minutes, or until lentils are tender.
5. Season: Adjust seasoning with salt and pepper to taste before serving.

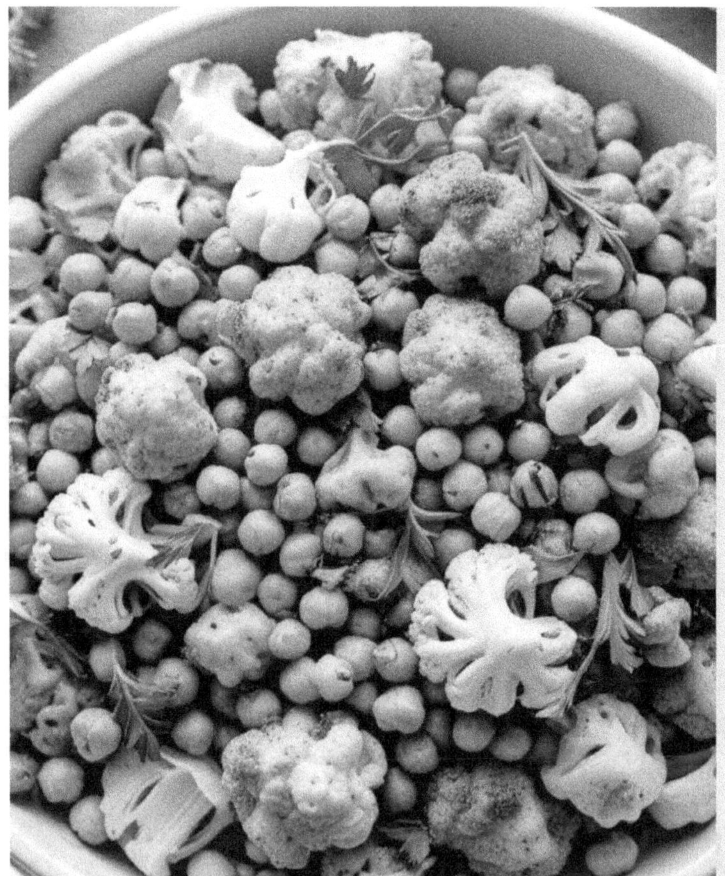

Roasted Cauliflower and Chickpeas

Prep Time	Cook Time

10 minutes	30 minutes

INGREDIENTS

- 1 head cauliflower, cut into florets
- 1 can (15 oz) chickpeas, drained and rinsed
- 2 tablespoons olive oil
- 1 teaspoon ground turmeric
- 1/2 teaspoon ground cumin
- 1/2 teaspoon smoked paprika
- Salt and pepper to taste

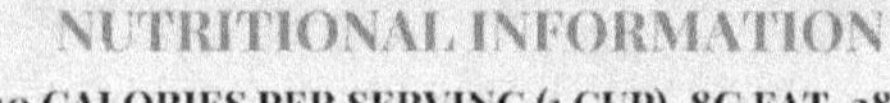

NUTRITIONAL INFORMATION

210 CALORIES PER SERVING (1 CUP), 8G FAT, 28G CARBOHYDRATES, 8G FIBER, 7G PROTEIN

DIRECTIONS

1. Preheat Oven: Preheat oven to 400°F (200°C).
2. Prepare Vegetables: In a large bowl, toss cauliflower florets and chickpeas with olive oil, turmeric, cumin, paprika, salt, and pepper.
3. Roast: Spread the mixture evenly on a baking sheet. Roast in the preheated oven for 25-30 minutes, or until cauliflower is golden brown and tender.
4. Serve: Enjoy warm as a side dish or over a bed of greens.

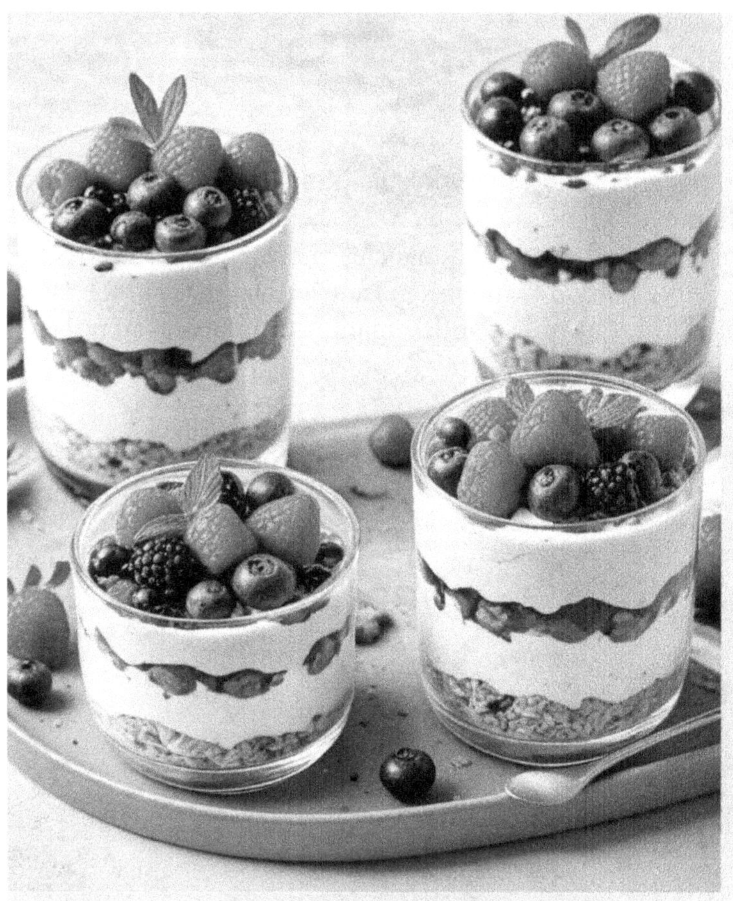

Greek Yogurt and Berry Parfait

Prep Time	Cook Time

10 minutes	0 minutes

INGREDIENTS

- 1 cup plain Greek yogurt
- 1/2 cup fresh mixed berries (strawberries, blueberries, raspberries)
- 2 tablespoons chia seeds
- 1 tablespoon honey or agave syrup (optional)
- 1/4 cup granola (optional)

NUTRITIONAL INFORMATION
180 CALORIES PER SERVING (1 CUP), 6G FAT, 20G
CARBOHYDRATES, 5G FIBER, 10G PROTEIN

DIRECTIONS

1. Prepare Chia Seeds: Stir chia seeds into Greek yogurt and let sit for 5 minutes to thicken.
2. Layer Parfait: In a glass or bowl, layer Greek yogurt mixture, fresh berries, and granola if using.
3. Sweeten: Drizzle honey or agave syrup over the top if desired.
4. Serve: Enjoy immediately or refrigerate for a chilled treat.

Anti-Inflammatory Meals

Meals containing anti-inflammatory components may be very helpful in managing and preventing cancer. Reducing chronic inflammation via nutrition may help reduce the risks associated with the development and progression of many malignancies. Leafy greens, berries, almonds, garlic, ginger, turmeric, and fatty fish are important anti-inflammatory foods. Antioxidants and substances that lessen oxidative stress and inflammation in the body may be found in abundance in these nutrients.

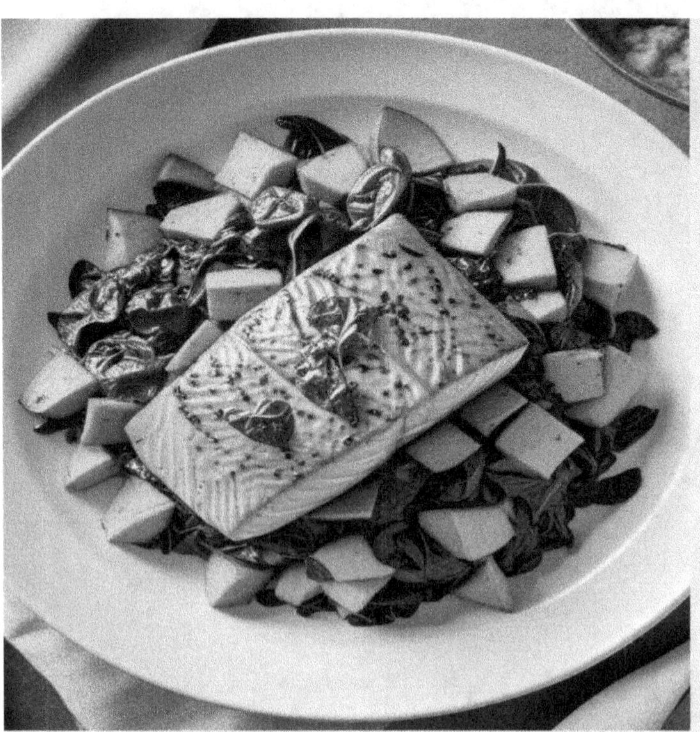

★★★★

Curried Salmon with Spinach and Sweet Potatoes

Prep Time
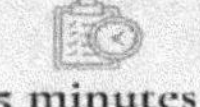
15 minutes

Cook Time
30 minutes

INGREDIENTS

- 4 salmon fillets
- 2 tablespoons olive oil
- 2 teaspoons ground turmeric
- 1 teaspoon ground cumin
- 1 teaspoon paprika
- 1/2 teaspoon black pepper
- 2 sweet potatoes, peeled and diced
- 3 cups fresh spinach
- 1 lemon, sliced

NUTRITIONAL INFORMATION
350 CALORIES PER SERVING, 20G FAT, 25G CARBOHYDRATES, 6G FIBER, 25G PROTEIN

DIRECTIONS

1. Preheat Oven: Preheat the oven to 400°F (200°C).
2. Season Salmon: Rub salmon fillets with olive oil, turmeric, cumin, paprika, and black pepper.
3. Prepare Sweet Potatoes: Spread diced sweet potatoes on a baking sheet, drizzle with a bit of olive oil, and season with salt and pepper. Roast for 20 minutes.
4. Cook Salmon: Place salmon fillets on the baking sheet with sweet potatoes and roast for an additional 15 minutes, or until the salmon is cooked through.
5. Add Spinach: Sauté spinach in a pan with a splash of olive oil until wilted. Serve salmon over the spinach with roasted sweet potatoes on the side.

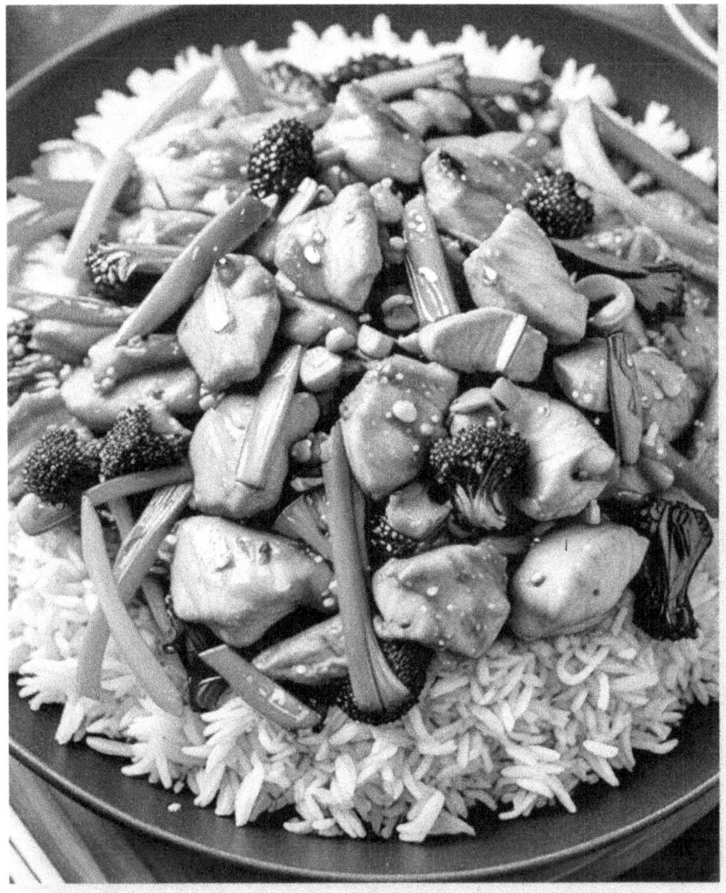

★★★★

Ginger-Garlic Chicken Stir-Fry

Prep Time

15 minutes

Cook Time

15 minutes

INGREDIENTS

- 1 lb chicken breast, sliced into strips
- 1 tablespoon olive oil
- 2 cloves garlic, minced
- 1-inch piece of fresh ginger, grated
- 2 bell peppers, sliced
- 1 cup broccoli florets
- 1 tablespoon tamari or soy sauce
- 1 tablespoon apple cider vinegar
- 1 tablespoon honey or agave syrup

DIRECTIONS

1. Heat Oil: In a large pan, heat olive oil over medium heat.
2. Cook Chicken: Add chicken strips and cook until browned and cooked through. Remove from pan and set aside.
3. Sauté Vegetables: In the same pan, add garlic and ginger, cooking for 1 minute. Add bell peppers and broccoli, stirring until vegetables are tender.
4. Combine: Return chicken to the pan. Stir in tamari, apple cider vinegar, and honey. Cook for an additional 2 minutes.
5. Serve: Serve hot, over brown rice or quinoa if desired.

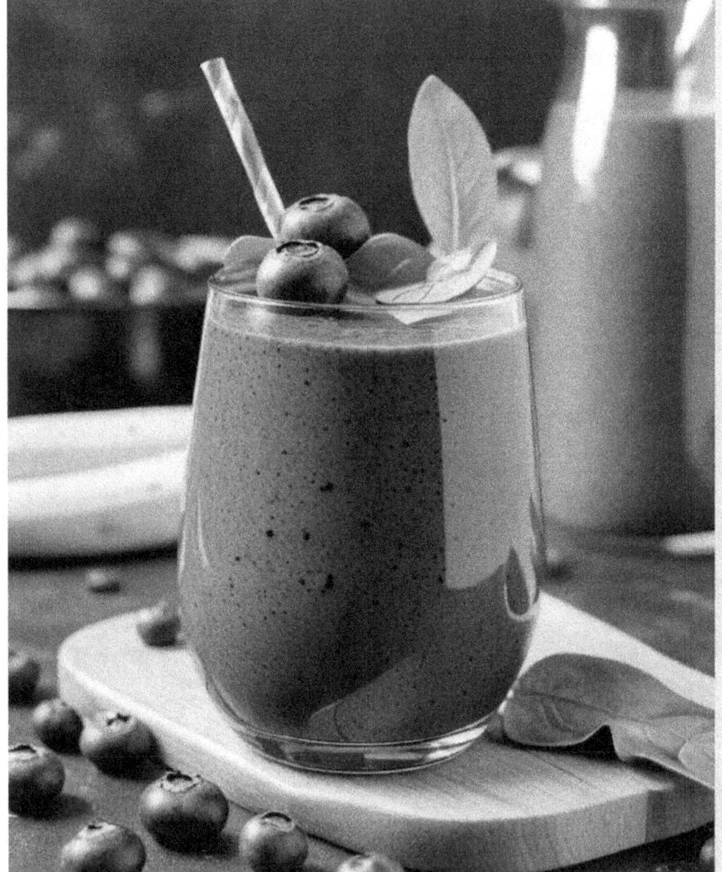

Blueberry and Spinach Smoothie

Prep Time

5 minutes

Cook Time

0 minutes

INGREDIENTS

- 1 cup fresh spinach leaves
- 1 cup frozen blueberries
- 1 banana
- 1 cup unsweetened almond milk
- 1 tablespoon chia seeds
- 1 tablespoon honey or maple syrup (optional)

NUTRITIONAL INFORMATION
220 CALORIES PER SERVING, 4G FAT, 36G CARBOHYDRATES, 7G FIBER, 5G PROTEIN

DIRECTIONS

1. Blend Ingredients: In a blender, combine spinach, blueberries, banana, almond milk, and chia seeds.
2. Sweeten: Add honey or maple syrup if additional sweetness is desired.
3. Blend: Blend until smooth and creamy.
4. Serve: Pour into a glass and enjoy immediately.

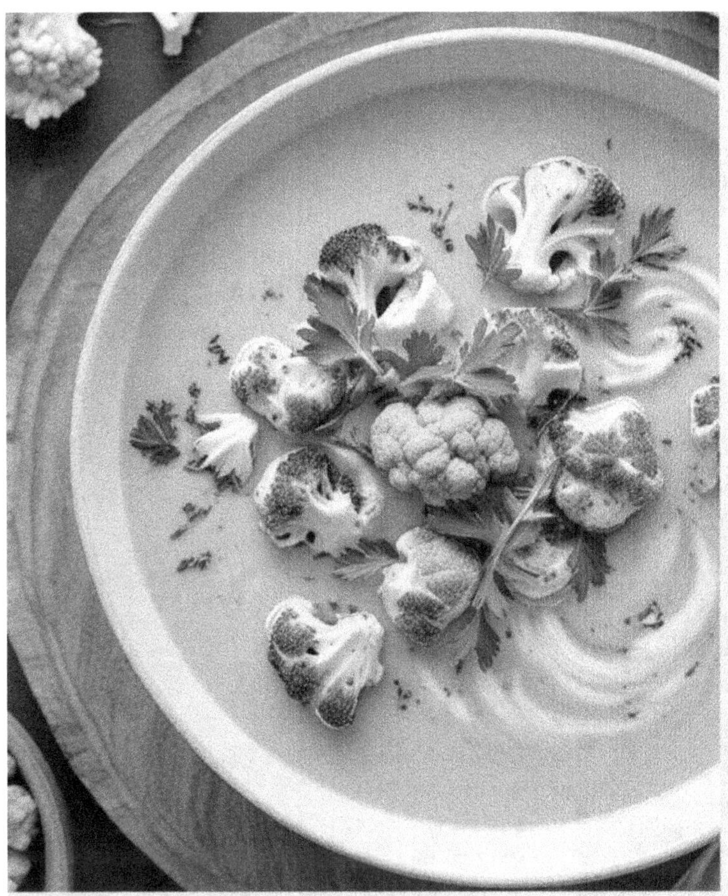

★★★★

Roasted Cauliflower and Turmeric Soup

Prep Time	Cook Time

15 minutes	35 minutes

INGREDIENTS

- 1 head cauliflower, cut into florets
- 2 tablespoons olive oil
- 1 teaspoon ground turmeric
- 1/2 teaspoon ground cumin
- 1/2 teaspoon smoked paprika
- 4 cups vegetable broth
- 1 onion, chopped
- 2 cloves garlic, minced
- Salt and pepper to taste

NUTRITIONAL INFORMATION

150 CALORIES PER SERVING (1 CUP), 7G FAT, 20G CARBOHYDRATES, 7G FIBER, 5G PROTEIN

DIRECTIONS

1. Preheat Oven: Preheat the oven to 400°F (200°C).
2. Roast Cauliflower: Toss cauliflower florets with olive oil, turmeric, cumin, paprika, salt, and pepper. Roast for 25 minutes, until tender and golden.
3. Sauté Vegetables: In a large pot, heat a splash of olive oil. Sauté onion and garlic until translucent.
4. Combine Ingredients: Add roasted cauliflower to the pot, pour in vegetable broth, and bring to a simmer for 10 minutes.
5. Blend Soup: Use an immersion blender or transfer to a blender to puree until smooth. Adjust seasoning as needed.

Gluten-Free Options

Making recipe modifications gluten-free doesn't have to mean sacrificing taste. Delicious recipes that satisfy dietary requirements without sacrificing flavor may be made by replacing gluten-containing items with gluten-free alternatives. Reducing inflammation and digestive problems associated with gluten sensitivity are among the advantages of a gluten-free diet for cancer care, which may also improve general health and well-being. Here are four delicious and fulfilling gluten-free recipes:

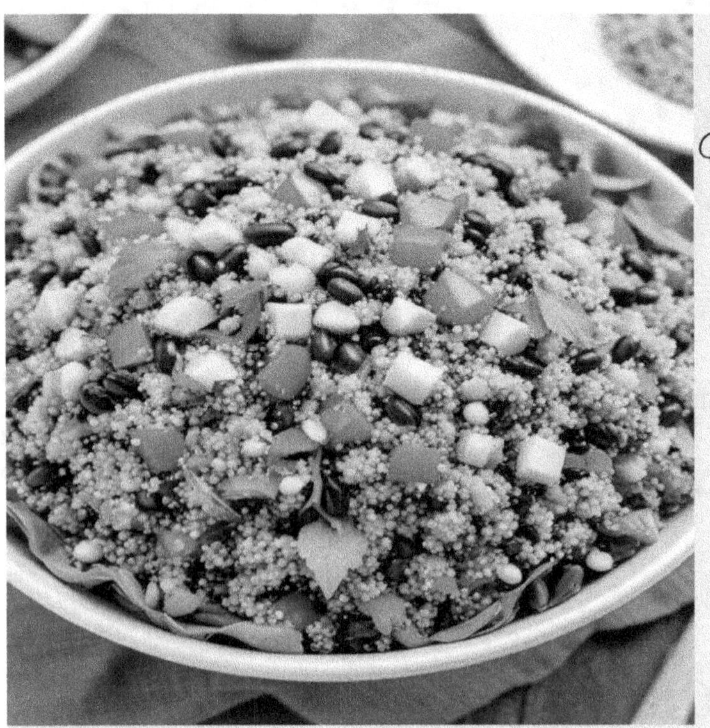

DIRECTIONS

1. Cook Quinoa: Rinse quinoa under cold water. In a medium saucepan, bring 2 cups of water to a boil. Add quinoa, reduce heat, cover, and simmer for 15 minutes. Remove from heat and let sit for 5 minutes, then fluff with a fork.
2. Combine Ingredients: In a large bowl, combine cooked quinoa, black beans, cherry tomatoes, red onion, and cilantro.
3. Dress Salad: Drizzle with lime juice and olive oil. Season with salt and pepper. Gently toss to combine.
4. Serve: Add diced avocado just before serving to keep it fresh.

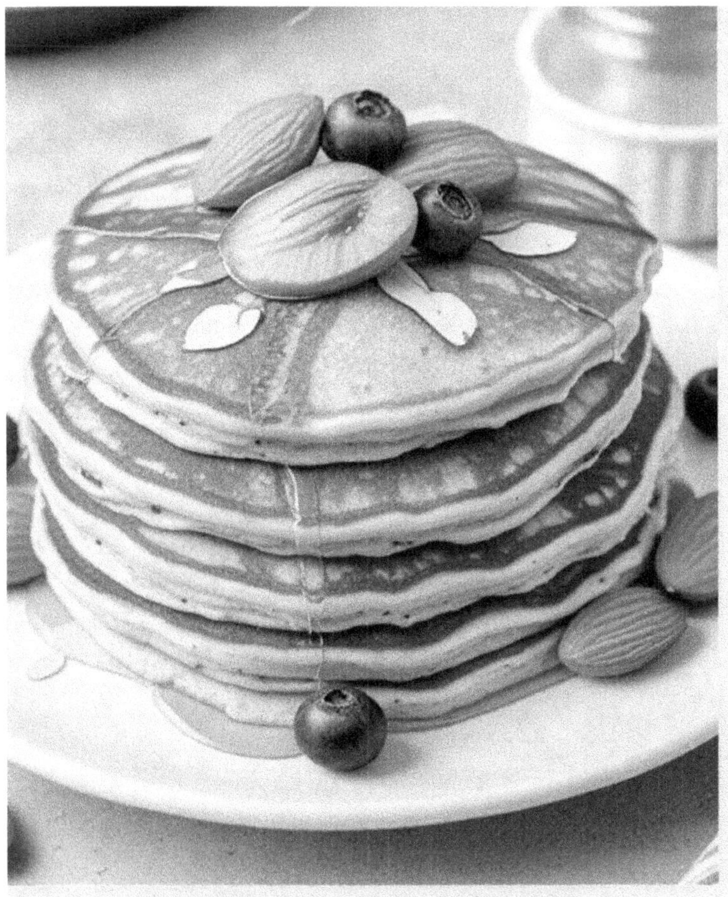

★★★★

Almond Flour Pancakes

Prep Time

10 minutes

Cook Time

10 minutes

INGREDIENTS

- 1 cup almond flour
- 2 large eggs
- 1/4 cup almond milk (or other non-dairy milk)
- 2 tablespoons honey or maple syrup
- 1 teaspoon vanilla extract
- 1/2 teaspoon baking soda
- Pinch of salt
- Butter or oil for cooking

NUTRITIONAL INFORMATION
200 CALORIES PER SERVING (2 PANCAKES), 14G
FAT, 12G CARBOHYDRATES, 3G FIBER, 8G PROTEIN

DIRECTIONS

1. Prepare Batter: In a bowl, whisk together almond flour, eggs, almond milk, honey, vanilla extract, baking soda, and salt until smooth.
2. Cook Pancakes: Heat a skillet over medium heat and add a small amount of butter or oil. Pour 1/4 cup of batter onto the skillet for each pancake. Cook until bubbles form on the surface, then flip and cook until golden brown.
3. Serve: Serve warm with your choice of toppings like fresh fruit, yogurt, or a drizzle of honey.

Sweet Potato and Chickpea Curry

Prep Time	Cook Time

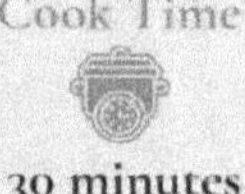

15 minutes   **30 minutes**

INGREDIENTS

- 2 medium sweet potatoes, peeled and diced
- 1 can chickpeas, drained and rinsed
- 1 can coconut milk
- 1 tablespoon olive oil
- 1 onion, chopped
- 2 cloves garlic, minced
- 1 tablespoon curry powder
- 1 teaspoon ground turmeric
- 1 teaspoon cumin
- Salt and pepper to taste
- Fresh cilantro for garnish

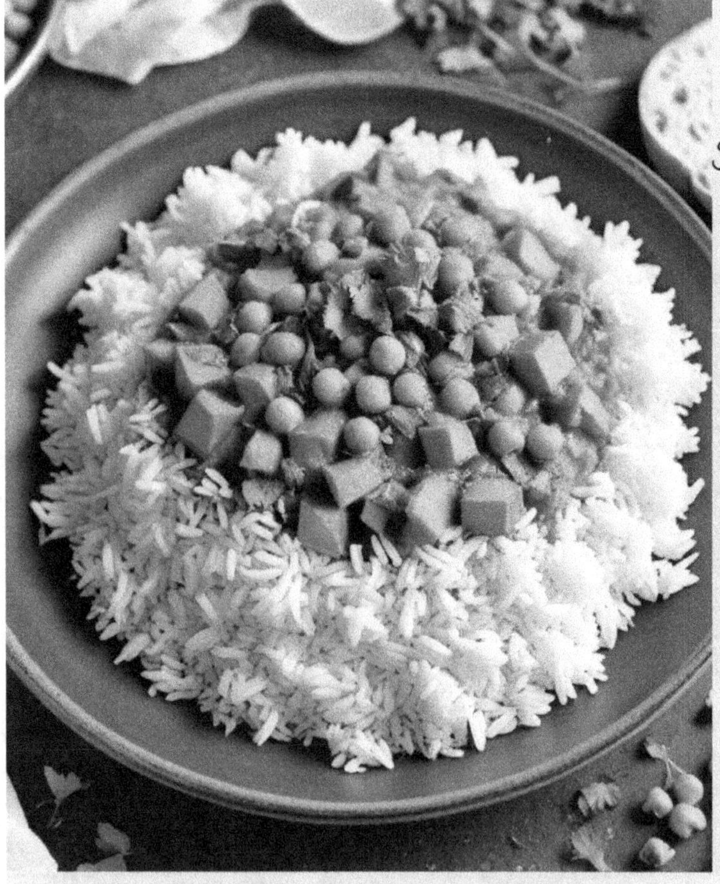

NUTRITIONAL INFORMATION

350 CALORIES PER SERVING, 20G FAT, 35G CARBOHYDRATES, 8G FIBER, 10G PROTEIN

DIRECTIONS

1. Cook Vegetables: Heat olive oil in a large pot over medium heat. Sauté onion and garlic until translucent. Add curry powder, turmeric, and cumin, stirring for 1 minute.
2. Add Sweet Potatoes: Add diced sweet potatoes and stir to coat with spices. Pour in coconut milk and bring to a simmer.
3. Simmer Curry: Cook for 15-20 minutes, until sweet potatoes are tender. Stir in chickpeas and cook for an additional 5 minutes.
4. Serve: Garnish with fresh cilantro before serving.

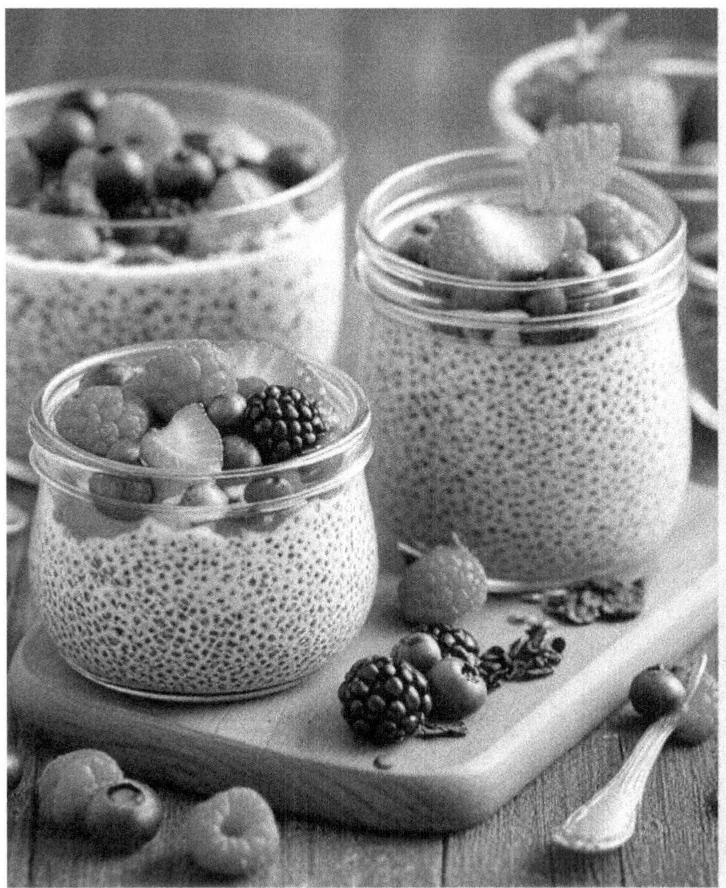

★★★★

Chia Seed Pudding with Fresh Berries

Prep Time
10 minutes

Cook Time
0 minutes

INGREDIENTS

- 1/4 cup chia seeds
- 1 cup unsweetened almond milk
- 1 tablespoon maple syrup or honey
- 1/2 teaspoon vanilla extract
- 1 cup mixed fresh berries (such as strawberries, blueberries, raspberries)

DIRECTIONS

1. Mix Pudding: In a bowl, whisk together chia seeds, almond milk, maple syrup, and vanilla extract. Let sit for 5 minutes, then stir again to ensure seeds are evenly distributed.
2. Refrigerate: Cover and refrigerate for at least 2 hours, or overnight, until the mixture has thickened to a pudding-like consistency.
3. Serve: Top with fresh berries before serving.

High Protein Plant-Based Recipes

Consuming enough protein is essential for those who are trying to control their cancer with a plant-based diet. Sources of plant-based protein provide the nutrients required for energy production, muscle maintenance, and general health. Hemp seeds, tofu, quinoa, lentils, and chickpeas are important sources of plant-based protein. You may satisfy your protein demands and get other vital nutrients by including them in your diet.

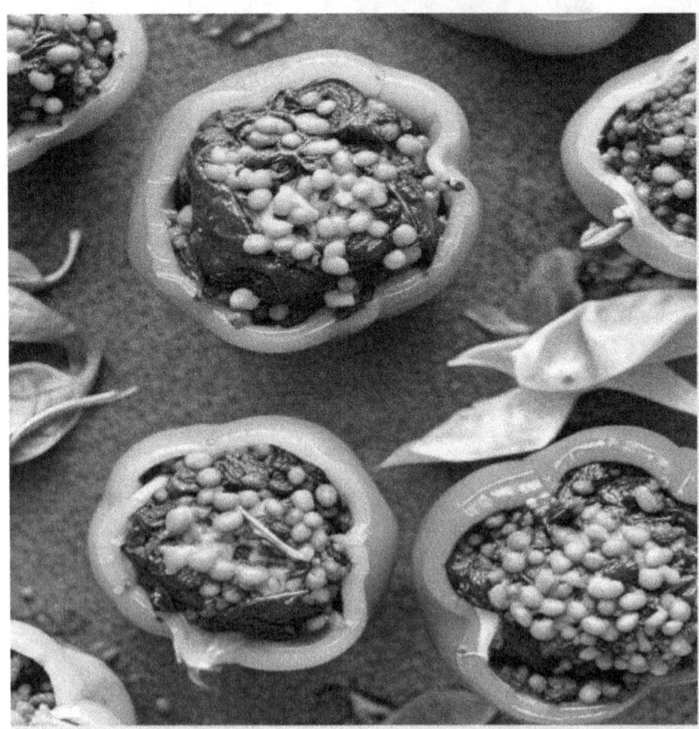

NUTRITIONAL INFORMATION
250 CALORIES PER SERVING, 6G FAT, 40G CARBOHYDRATES, 10G FIBER, 12G PROTEIN

INGREDIENTS

- 4 large bell peppers
- 1 cup cooked green lentils
- 1 cup cooked quinoa
- 1 cup fresh spinach, chopped
- 1/2 cup diced tomatoes
- 1/2 cup finely chopped onion
- 2 cloves garlic, minced
- 1 tablespoon olive oil
- 1 teaspoon cumin
- Salt and pepper to taste
- Fresh cilantro for garnish

DIRECTIONS

1. Prepare Peppers: Preheat oven to 375°F (190°C). Cut the tops off the bell peppers and remove seeds. Place in a baking dish.
2. Cook Filling: In a pan, heat olive oil over medium heat. Sauté onion and garlic until translucent. Add diced tomatoes, cumin, salt, and pepper. Stir in cooked lentils, quinoa, and spinach. Cook until spinach is wilted.
3. Stuff Peppers: Fill each bell pepper with the lentil mixture. Cover with foil and bake for 30 minutes. Remove foil and bake for an additional 10 minutes.
4. Serve: Garnish with fresh cilantro before serving.

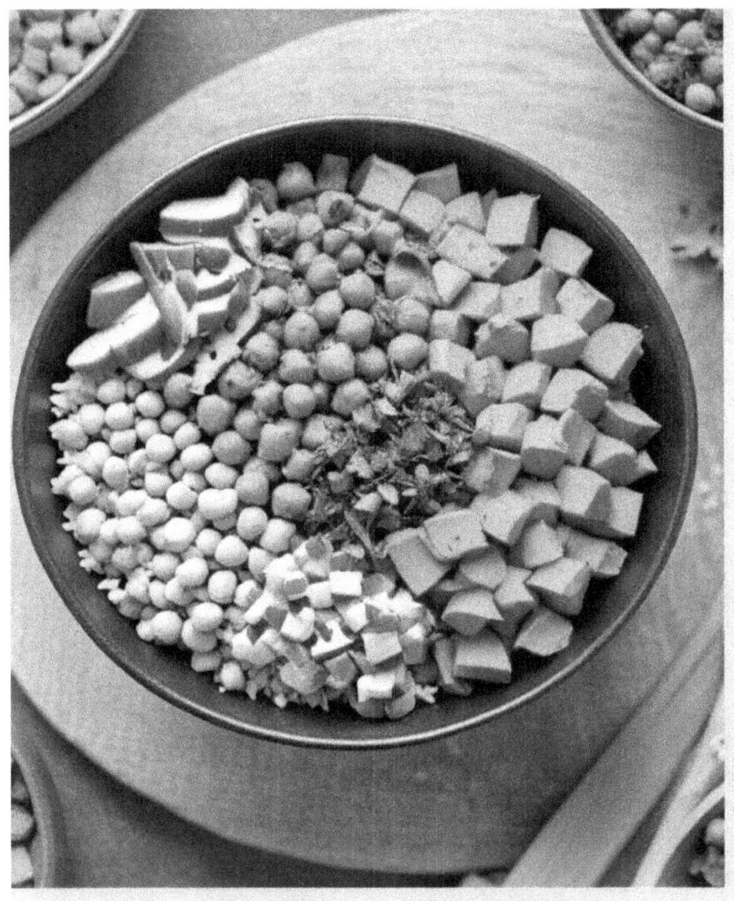

Spicy Chickpea and Sweet Potato Bowl

Prep Time	Cook Time

15 minutes   30 minutes

INGREDIENTS

- 1 can chickpeas, drained and rinsed
- 2 medium sweet potatoes, peeled and cubed
- 2 tablespoons olive oil
- 1 teaspoon smoked paprika
- 1/2 teaspoon cayenne pepper
- 1 teaspoon garlic powder
- Salt and pepper to taste
- 2 cups kale, chopped
- 1 avocado, sliced

NUTRITIONAL INFORMATION
400 CALORIES PER SERVING, 15G FAT, 50G CARBOHYDRATES, 10G FIBER, 15G PROTEIN

DIRECTIONS

1. Prepare Vegetables: Preheat oven to 400°F (200°C). Toss sweet potato cubes with olive oil, smoked paprika, cayenne pepper, garlic powder, salt, and pepper. Spread on a baking sheet and roast for 25-30 minutes until tender.
2. Cook Chickpeas: On a separate baking sheet, toss chickpeas with a bit of olive oil, salt, and pepper. Roast for 15-20 minutes until crispy.
3. Assemble Bowl: In a bowl, combine roasted sweet potatoes, crispy chickpeas, and chopped kale. Top with avocado slices.
4. Serve: Enjoy warm or at room temperature.

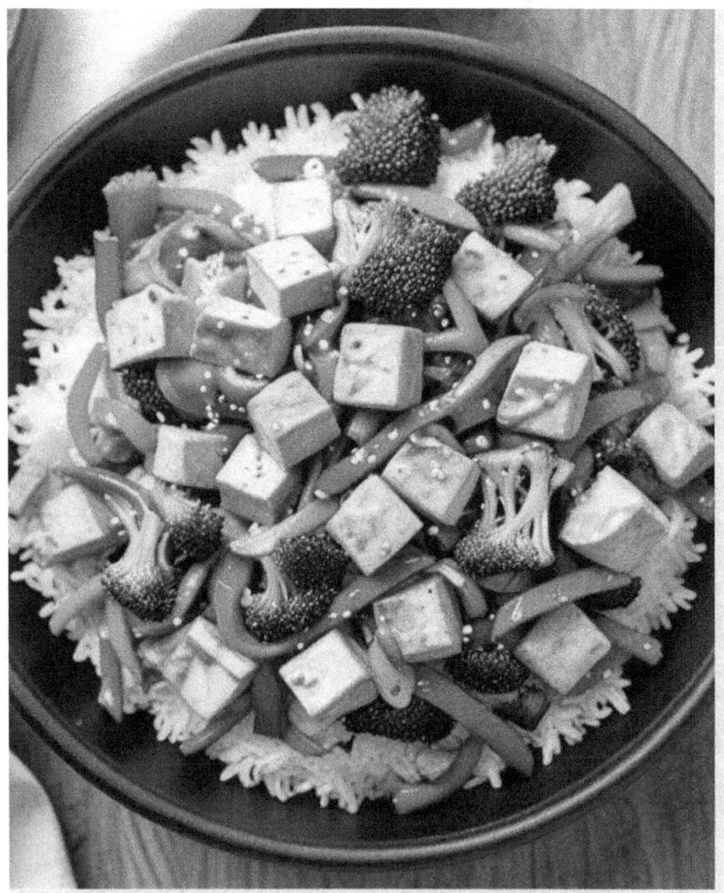

★★★★

Tofu and Vegetable Stir-Fry

Prep Time

15 minutes

Cook Time

15 minutes

INGREDIENTS

- 1 block firm tofu, drained and cubed
- 1 tablespoon soy sauce
- 1 tablespoon sesame oil
- 1 cup broccoli florets
- 1 cup bell peppers, sliced
- 1 cup snap peas
- 2 cloves garlic, minced
- 1 tablespoon grated ginger
- 2 tablespoons hoisin sauce
- 1 tablespoon sesame seeds

NUTRITIONAL INFORMATION

300 CALORIES PER SERVING, 15G FAT, 20G CARBOHYDRATES, 5G FIBER, 20G PROTEIN

DIRECTIONS

1. Prepare Tofu: Heat sesame oil in a pan over medium heat. Add cubed tofu and cook until golden brown on all sides. Remove from pan and set aside.
2. Stir-Fry Vegetables: In the same pan, add garlic and ginger, and cook until fragrant. Add broccoli, bell peppers, and snap peas. Stir-fry until tender-crisp.
3. Combine Ingredients: Return tofu to the pan. Add soy sauce and hoisin sauce, tossing to coat evenly. Cook for an additional 2 minutes.
4. Serve: Garnish with sesame seeds before serving.

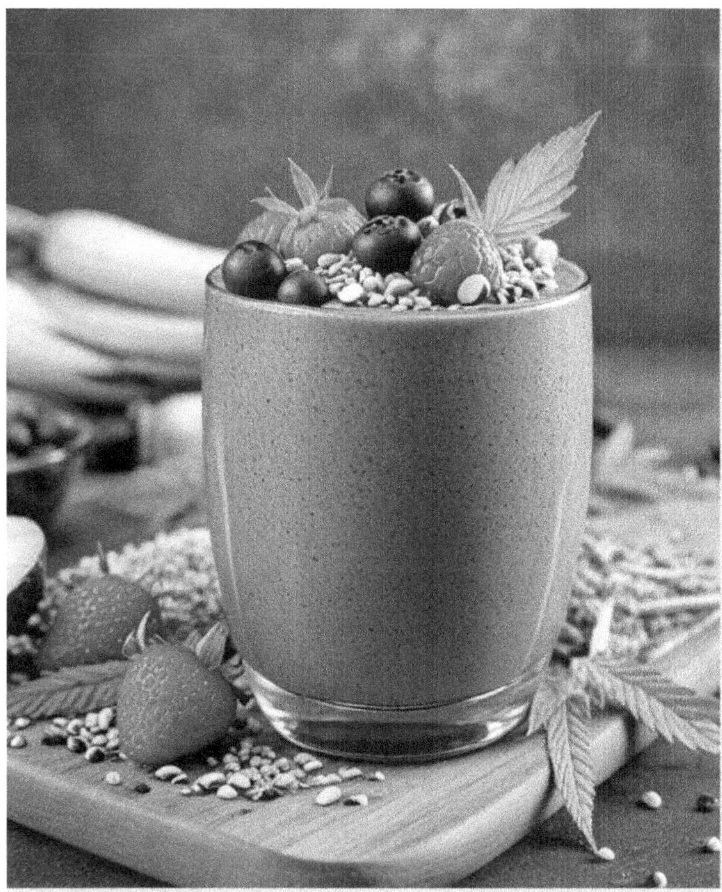

Hemp Seed and Berry Smoothie

Prep Time

5 minutes

Cook Time

5 minutes

INGREDIENTS

- 1 cup unsweetened almond milk
- 1/2 cup frozen mixed berries
- 2 tablespoons hemp seeds
- 1 tablespoon chia seeds
- 1 banana
- 1 tablespoon maple syrup (optional)

NUTRITIONAL INFORMATION
250 CALORIES PER SERVING, 10G FAT, 30G
CARBOHYDRATES, 8G FIBER, 10G PROTEIN

DIRECTIONS

1. Blend Ingredients: In a blender, combine almond milk, frozen berries, hemp seeds, chia seeds, and banana. Blend until smooth.
2. Adjust Sweetness: Taste and add maple syrup if desired. Blend again.
3. Serve: Pour into a glass and enjoy immediately.

CHAPTER 10

Meal Plans and Prep Guides

30-Day Cancer Prevention Meal Plan

This 30-day meal plan has a carefully curated mix of nutrient-dense, plant-based meals that are intended to assist cancer prevention. Every meal is designed to include components that are recognized for their ability to combat cancer, offering a nutritious and well-balanced diet that supports optimum health.

A range of foods high in antioxidants, vitamins, minerals, and phytonutrients are highlighted in the meal plan. Breakfast alternatives that are high in fruits, vegetables, and seeds that are believed to reduce oxidative stress include the Antioxidant Berry Oatmeal and the Green Smoothie Power Bowl. These components boost immunity and promote cellular health, both of which are essential for preventing cancer. For a more varied and nutrient-dense start to each day, try the Sweet Potato and Black Bean Breakfast Burrito and Chia Seed Pudding with Fresh Fruit.

Lunch options include high-fiber and plant-based protein meals like lentil and spinach soup quinoa and roasted vegetable salad. A complete protein, quinoa has important amino acids that support general health. Vegetables retain their nutritional value and take on a richer taste when they are roasted, which contributes to the health benefits of dishes like Raw Rainbow Vegetable Noodle Salad and Mediterranean Chickpea Wrap.

The menu calls for hearty dishes like stuffed bell peppers with cauliflower rice and spaghetti squash with tomato basil sauce for supper. Low-calorie spaghetti squash may be substituted for pasta, and tomatoes and basil together provide an abundant supply of lycopene, an antioxidant associated with a decreased risk of cancer. Since broccoli is renowned for its sulforaphane content, which has been examined for its anti-cancer benefits, and tofu is a significant source of plant-based protein, Tofu Stir-Fry with Broccoli and Cashews offers a substantial dinner with cancer-fighting characteristics.

A range of filling appetizers and sweets, such as Dark Chocolate Avocado Mousse and Spicy Roasted Chickpeas, are also included in the plan. Dark Chocolate Avocado Mousse is a rich, creamy delight full of antioxidants and good fats, while Spicy Roasted Chickpeas give a crunchy, high-protein snack that helps control blood sugar and hunger. These snacks help maintain a balanced food intake in addition to staving off hunger.

You will gain from a methodical approach to meal preparation by adhering to this scheduled meal plan. The plan makes sure that meals are nutrient-dense and diverse, which helps keep things interesting and encourages following a diet that lowers the risk of cancer. Moreover, organized meal planning lowers food waste, promotes healthier grocery shopping practices, and expedites daily meal preparation.

Apart from its pragmatic advantages, this methodology aids in maintaining a steady consumption of essential nutrients that promote cancer avoidance. A variety of fruits, vegetables, whole grains, legumes, and nuts are included in each meal to guarantee a thorough consumption of vital nutrients. This variety offers a wide range of phytonutrients and antioxidants, maximizing the health advantages of the diet.

The 30-day meal plan is intended to promote general health and well-being in addition to cancer prevention. It helps guarantee that all nutritional demands are satisfied while encouraging a lifestyle that may lower the risk of chronic illnesses by combining a wide variety of plant-based meals. Adhering to a regimented meal plan such as this one is a useful, efficient approach to maintaining a nutritious diet and making knowledgeable food decisions.

Weekly Meal Prep Tips and Strategies

You may turn your daily plant-based eating regimen into a simplified, stress-free procedure by meal planning. The secret is to organize and prepare ahead so that eating a healthy diet may be both fun and doable. Here are some tips to help you maximize meal prep and incorporate it easily into your weekly schedule.

To begin, schedule a certain time each week to prepare meals. Selecting a day, such as Sunday or Wednesday, facilitates the establishment of a habit. Make sure to concentrate on cooking basic components during this period instead of whole meals. Prepare large quantities of basic foods like grains, beans, and roasted veggies so you can utilize them in different dishes all week long. For example, a large batch of brown rice or quinoa may be used as the foundation for bowls, stir-fries, and salads.

Set up your kitchen to facilitate effective meal preparation. Make sure you have the appropriate equipment, including measuring cups, storage containers, cutting boards, and sharp blades. Purchasing airtight, high-quality containers can help your food stay fresher for longer and avoid spoiling. Meal planning is made simpler because ready items can be easily seen within clear glass containers, which are great for storing them. To meet varying portion requirements, think about offering a range of sizes.

Making a meal plan in advance can make preparation much easier. Based on the meals you want to make, make a weekly menu and shopping list. By doing this, you may minimize food waste and avoid making impulsive purchases while also making sure you have all the ingredients on hand. To manage your shopping lists, prep schedules, and meal plans, use an easy spreadsheet or an app. This gives a clear weekly schedule and helps in visualizing the tasks that need to be completed.

Batch cooking is a potent tactic for effective meal preparation. Make a lot of different ingredients that work well together and can be used in many recipes. For instance, cook a pot of lentils, roast a large tray of veggies, and make a large quantity of your preferred dressing. You may combine them to make a variety of meals. Grain-free cooked beans and roasted vegetables may be frozen for extended storage, or they can be kept in the refrigerator for up to a week. This method allows for flexibility in meal preparation in addition to time savings.

When it comes to actually preparing the meals, begin with the chores that take the longest. For example, start roasting veggies early so you can do other things while they're cooking. Chop all of your veggies and put them in storage containers. If you're cooking dishes that will last longer, you can even freeze them. To give your food more taste and diversity, make marinades, dressings, and sauces ahead of time. Having these ingredients ready to go can speed up and improve the experience of making meals.

To make meals interesting, think about combining different cooking techniques. Use a variety of cooking methods, like baking, grilling, and steaming, to vary up your preparation. For example, you may steam greens on the stovetop and roast other veggies in the oven at the same time. This maintains your food' variety of textures while also enhancing taste.

Another crucial component of meal preparation is portion management. Separating your prepared items into small servings facilitates quick meal-on-the-go eating and aids in calorie management. When preparing meals that are well-balanced and include grains, veggies, and protein, using containers with parts may be very helpful. By following this routine, you may avoid overeating and make sure that every meal contains a range of nutrients.

Lastly, have fun with meal planning by experimenting with different tastes and dishes. Using a variety of herbs, spices, and sauces can keep your dishes interesting and avoid becoming boring. Change up your meal selections often to include a range of nutrients and prevent diet boredom. Rather than being a hassle, meal preparation ought to be a fulfilling aspect of your week.

Meal planning may become a natural and manageable part of your weekly schedule by implementing these methods into your routine. It turns the procedure from a difficult undertaking into a productive, well-organized routine that promotes a plant-based, healthful lifestyle.

Batch Cooking and Freezing Guidelines

For those who want to keep their diet healthful while simplifying meal preparation, batch cooking, and freezing work well. By setting aside time to prepare big amounts of food and freeze it correctly, you may build up a pantry of wholesome, prepared meals that make eating healthily simple and easy.

Planning your menu and choosing recipes that are both adaptable and freezer-friendly is the first step in bulk cooking. Go for meals like soups, stews, casseroles, and grain-based recipes that keep their taste and texture even after being frozen and reheated. When reheated, recipes that strike a balance between protein, veggies, and healthy grains tend to store well and provide satisfying dinners.

For batch cooking to be effective, preparation is essential. Arrange your kitchen first, then collect all the supplies and equipment you'll need. Make a freezer-safe investment in high-grade storage containers. To avoid freezer burn and maintain the quality of the food, choose airtight containers made of glass or BPA-free plastic. , resealable freezer bags are great for saving space, especially when used for products like sauces and soups.

Efficiency is key when cooking in large quantities. Cook specific ingredients in huge quantities so they may be used in other recipes. For example, make a ton of beans, roast several trays of mixed veggies, and prepare a huge pot of quinoa or brown rice. These ingredients may be mixed and matched to make a variety of dishes. This method guarantees that you have a range of alternatives accessible while also saving you time.

Following cooking, using the right freezing methods is crucial to preserving the quality of your food. Transfer the meal to the freezer after letting it cool to room temperature. The temperature within your freezer may rise due to hot food, which might compromise the quality of other products. Before freezing, divide the food into portions the size of a meal. By following this procedure, you may save waste and only thaw what you need. To keep track of what you have and prevent misunderstanding, label each container with the date and contents.

Freezing is a great method to keep your food's nutritious content intact. When frozen, the majority of plant-based foods, including grains and vegetables, maintain their vitamin and mineral content. It's crucial to remember that not all substances freeze properly. For instance, after freezing, foods rich in water content, such as salads or meals with a lot of dairy replacements, may become mushy or lose texture. As a result, choose recipes carefully and take into account how the components will freeze.

To guarantee even heating and preserve texture, reheat frozen meals gradually. If you're pressed for time, you may defrost your food in your microwave or thaw it overnight in the refrigerator. To guarantee safety, fully reheat to an internal temperature of 165°F (74°C). Reheating some foods, such as soups and stews, could benefit from a brief stir to disperse the flavors and heat.

Cooking in batches has a lot of time savings advantages. You may cut down on the amount of time you spend cooking on hectic days by prepping meals in advance. , it reduces the need for poor food choices or last-minute takeout, promoting a balanced diet. Having a well-stocked freezer allows you to always have a wholesome meal available, which may support your commitment to a plant-based diet and healthy eating objectives.

Bulk cooking may be an affordable method of controlling your food spending. The cost per serving is often lower when components are purchased in bigger amounts. You may manage the quality and nutritional value of your food while saving money by cooking at home instead of purchasing prepackaged or eating out.

Including freezing and batch cooking in your routine helps you live a healthy lifestyle in addition to streamlining the process of preparing meals. Efficient meal planning, preparation, and storage guarantees that you always have easy access to nutrient-dense foods, which makes it simpler to maintain a plant-based, balanced diet and adhere to dietary objectives.

Week 1

Day 1:

- **Breakfast:** Green Smoothie Power Bowl
- **Lunch:** Quinoa and Roasted Vegetable Salad
- **Dinner:** Spaghetti Squash with Tomato Basil Sauce
- **Snack:** Spicy Roasted Chickpeas
- **Dessert:** Dark Chocolate Avocado Mousse

Day 2:

- **Breakfast:** Antioxidant Berry Oatmeal
- **Lunch:** Lentil and Spinach Soup
- **Dinner:** Stuffed Bell Peppers with Cauliflower Rice
- **Snack:** Almond and Date Energy Balls
- **Dessert:** Berry Chia Jam with Almond Butter

Day 3:

- **Breakfast:** Sweet Potato and Black Bean Breakfast Burrito
- **Lunch:** Mediterranean Chickpea Wrap
- **Dinner:** Tofu Stir-Fry with Broccoli and Cashews
- **Snack:** Veggie Sticks with Hummus
- **Dessert:** Apple Cinnamon Crumble

Day 4:

- **Breakfast:** Chia Seed Pudding with Fresh Fruit
- **Lunch:** Raw Rainbow Vegetable Noodle Salad
- **Dinner:** Sweet and Spicy Butternut Squash Curry
- **Snack:** Baked Kale Chips
- **Dessert:** Coconut Mango Sorbet

Day 5:

- **Breakfast:** Green Smoothie Power Bowl
- **Lunch:** Quinoa and Roasted Vegetable Salad
- **Dinner:** Spaghetti Squash with Tomato Basil Sauce
- **Snack:** Spicy Roasted Chickpeas
- **Dessert:** Dark Chocolate Avocado Mousse

Day 6:

- **Breakfast:** Antioxidant Berry Oatmeal
- **Lunch:** Lentil and Spinach Soup
- **Dinner:** Stuffed Bell Peppers with Cauliflower Rice
- **Snack:** Almond and Date Energy Balls
- **Dessert:** Berry Chia Jam with Almond Butter

Day 7:

- **Breakfast:** Sweet Potato and Black Bean Breakfast Burrito
- **Lunch:** Mediterranean Chickpea Wrap
- **Dinner:** Tofu Stir-Fry with Broccoli and Cashews
- **Snack:** Veggie Sticks with Hummus
- **Dessert:** Apple Cinnamon Crumble

Week 2

Day 8:

- **Breakfast:** Chia Seed Pudding with Fresh Fruit
- **Lunch:** Raw Rainbow Vegetable Noodle Salad

- **Dinner:** Sweet and Spicy Butternut Squash Curry
- **Snack:** Baked Kale Chips
- **Dessert:** Coconut Mango Sorbet

Day 9:

- **Breakfast:** Green Smoothie Power Bowl
- **Lunch:** Quinoa and Roasted Vegetable Salad
- **Dinner:** Spaghetti Squash with Tomato Basil Sauce
- **Snack:** Spicy Roasted Chickpeas
- **Dessert:** Dark Chocolate Avocado Mousse

Day 10:

- **Breakfast:** Antioxidant Berry Oatmeal
- **Lunch:** Lentil and Spinach Soup
- **Dinner:** Stuffed Bell Peppers with Cauliflower Rice
- **Snack:** Almond and Date Energy Balls
- **Dessert:** Berry Chia Jam with Almond Butter

Day 11:

- **Breakfast:** Sweet Potato and Black Bean Breakfast Burrito
- **Lunch:** Mediterranean Chickpea Wrap
- **Dinner:** Tofu Stir-Fry with Broccoli and Cashews
- **Snack:** Veggie Sticks with Hummus
- **Dessert:** Apple Cinnamon Crumble

Day 12:

- **Breakfast:** Chia Seed Pudding with Fresh Fruit
- **Lunch:** Raw Rainbow Vegetable Noodle Salad

- **Dinner:** Sweet and Spicy Butternut Squash Curry
- **Snack:** Baked Kale Chips
- **Dessert:** Coconut Mango Sorbet

Day 13:

- **Breakfast:** Green Smoothie Power Bowl
- **Lunch:** Quinoa and Roasted Vegetable Salad
- **Dinner:** Spaghetti Squash with Tomato Basil Sauce
- **Snack:** Spicy Roasted Chickpeas
- **Dessert:** Dark Chocolate Avocado Mousse

Day 14:

- **Breakfast:** Antioxidant Berry Oatmeal
- **Lunch:** Lentil and Spinach Soup
- **Dinner:** Stuffed Bell Peppers with Cauliflower Rice
- **Snack:** Almond and Date Energy Balls
- **Dessert:** Berry Chia Jam with Almond Butter

Week 3

Day 15:

- **Breakfast:** Sweet Potato and Black Bean Breakfast Burrito
- **Lunch:** Mediterranean Chickpea Wrap
- **Dinner:** Tofu Stir-Fry with Broccoli and Cashews
- **Snack:** Veggie Sticks with Hummus
- **Dessert:** Apple Cinnamon Crumble

Day 16:

- **Breakfast:** Chia Seed Pudding with Fresh Fruit

- **Lunch:** Raw Rainbow Vegetable Noodle Salad
- **Dinner:** Sweet and Spicy Butternut Squash Curry
- **Snack:** Baked Kale Chips
- **Dessert:** Coconut Mango Sorbet

Day 17:

- **Breakfast:** Green Smoothie Power Bowl
- **Lunch:** Quinoa and Roasted Vegetable Salad
- **Dinner:** Spaghetti Squash with Tomato Basil Sauce
- **Snack:** Spicy Roasted Chickpeas
- **Dessert:** Dark Chocolate Avocado Mousse

Day 18:

- **Breakfast:** Antioxidant Berry Oatmeal
- **Lunch:** Lentil and Spinach Soup
- **Dinner:** Stuffed Bell Peppers with Cauliflower Rice
- **Snack:** Almond and Date Energy Balls
- **Dessert:** Berry Chia Jam with Almond Butter

Day 19:

- **Breakfast:** Sweet Potato and Black Bean Breakfast Burrito
- **Lunch:** Mediterranean Chickpea Wrap
- **Dinner:** Tofu Stir-Fry with Broccoli and Cashews
- **Snack:** Veggie Sticks with Hummus
- **Dessert:** Apple Cinnamon Crumble

Day 20:

- **Breakfast:** Chia Seed Pudding with Fresh Fruit

- **Lunch:** Raw Rainbow Vegetable Noodle Salad
- **Dinner:** Sweet and Spicy Butternut Squash Curry
- **Snack:** Baked Kale Chips
- **Dessert:** Coconut Mango Sorbet

Day 21:

- **Breakfast:** Green Smoothie Power Bowl
- **Lunch:** Quinoa and Roasted Vegetable Salad
- **Dinner:** Spaghetti Squash with Tomato Basil Sauce
- **Snack:** Spicy Roasted Chickpeas
- **Dessert:** Dark Chocolate Avocado Mousse

Week 4

Day 22:

- **Breakfast:** Antioxidant Berry Oatmeal
- **Lunch:** Lentil and Spinach Soup
- **Dinner:** Stuffed Bell Peppers with Cauliflower Rice
- **Snack:** Almond and Date Energy Balls
- **Dessert:** Berry Chia Jam with Almond Butter

Day 23:

- **Breakfast:** Sweet Potato and Black Bean Breakfast Burrito
- **Lunch:** Mediterranean Chickpea Wrap
- **Dinner:** Tofu Stir-Fry with Broccoli and Cashews
- **Snack:** Veggie Sticks with Hummus
- **Dessert:** Apple Cinnamon Crumble

Day 24:

- **Breakfast:** Chia Seed Pudding with Fresh Fruit
- **Lunch:** Raw Rainbow Vegetable Noodle Salad
- **Dinner:** Sweet and Spicy Butternut Squash Curry
- **Snack:** Baked Kale Chips
- **Dessert:** Coconut Mango Sorbet

Day 25:

- **Breakfast:** Green Smoothie Power Bowl
- **Lunch:** Quinoa and Roasted Vegetable Salad
- **Dinner:** Spaghetti Squash with Tomato Basil Sauce
- **Snack:** Spicy Roasted Chickpeas
- **Dessert:** Dark Chocolate Avocado Mousse

Day 26:

- **Breakfast:** Antioxidant Berry Oatmeal
- **Lunch:** Lentil and Spinach Soup
- **Dinner:** Stuffed Bell Peppers with Cauliflower Rice
- **Snack:** Almond and Date Energy Balls
- **Dessert:** Berry Chia Jam with Almond Butter

Day 27:

- **Breakfast:** Sweet Potato and Black Bean Breakfast Burrito
- **Lunch:** Mediterranean Chickpea Wrap

- **Dinner:** Tofu Stir-Fry with Broccoli and Cashews
- **Snack:** Veggie Sticks with Hummus
- **Dessert:** Apple Cinnamon Crumble

Day 28:

- **Breakfast:** Chia Seed Pudding with Fresh Fruit
- **Lunch:** Raw Rainbow Vegetable Noodle Salad
- **Dinner:** Sweet and Spicy Butternut Squash Curry
- **Snack:** Baked Kale Chips
- **Dessert:** Coconut Mango Sorbet

Day 29:

- **Breakfast:** Green Smoothie Power Bowl
- **Lunch:** Quinoa and Roasted Vegetable Salad
- **Dinner:** Spaghetti Squash with Tomato Basil Sauce
- **Snack:** Spicy Roasted Chickpeas
- **Dessert:** Dark Chocolate Avocado Mousse

Day 30:

- **Breakfast:** Antioxidant Berry Oatmeal
- **Lunch:** Lentil and Spinach Soup
- **Dinner:** Stuffed Bell Peppers with Cauliflower Rice
- **Snack:** Almond and Date Energy Balls
- **Dessert:** Berry Chia Jam with Almond Butter

APPENDICES

Nutritional Information for Key Ingredients

Knowing the nutritional makeup of important substances may greatly improve your capacity to make well-informed dietary decisions, particularly when trying to promote general health and cancer prevention. You may customize your diet to optimize its health advantages and meet your objectives by concentrating on certain nutrients and their functions in the body.

Understanding the role of antioxidants in food is essential to making wise decisions. These substances aid in the body's elimination of free radicals, which might lessen inflammation and oxidative stress—factors associated with the development of cancer. Berries, leafy greens, and nuts are among the ingredients high in antioxidants. For example, berries are a great source of flavonoids and vitamins C and E, which have been shown to enhance immune system function and prevent cell damage. Leafy greens such as kale and spinach are rich in lutein (linked to a decreased risk of cancer) and vitamin K (important in cell development and apoptosis). Nuts, especially walnuts and almonds, provide vitamin E and good fats that support cellular health and lower inflammation.

Another vital factor in substances that combat cancer is fiber. Encouraging regular bowel movements helps maintain digestive health and may help reduce the risk of colorectal cancer. Good sources of dietary fiber include vegetables, legumes, and whole grains. Quinoa, for instance, offers a substantial quantity of fiber that promotes satiety and digestion in addition to serving as a complete protein source. Both beans and lentils have a high fiber content and provide other advantages like protein and important minerals like magnesium and iron.

The natural substances included in plants, known as phytonutrients, are also essential in preventing cancer. These include glucosinolates, which are present in cruciferous vegetables like broccoli and Brussels sprouts, and carotenoids, which are found in orange and yellow foods like sweet potatoes and carrots. Beta-carotene is one of the carotenoids that may be transformed into vitamin A, which is necessary for the mucous membranes and skin to remain healthy. It has been shown that glucosinolates aid in the body's detoxification activities and may prevent the spread of cancer cells.

Apart from phytonutrients, fiber, and antioxidants, good fats are essential for general well-being and may have an impact on cancer prevention. Nuts, seeds, and avocados are sources of good fats. Avocados are a great source of monounsaturated fats, which are important for maintaining cell membrane integrity and heart health. Omega-3 fatty acids, which have anti-inflammatory qualities and may help lower the risk of several malignancies, are abundant in seeds, especially chia and flaxseeds.

It takes more than simply smart food selection to include essential nutrients in your diet. It also entails knowing how to mix and prepare them to get the most out of them. For instance, boiling tomatoes may make lycopene, a strong antioxidant that may lower the risk of prostate cancer, more bioavailable. Likewise, combining foods high in iron, such as spinach, with foods high in vitamin C, such as citrus fruits, may improve iron absorption and promote general health and well-being.

When making dietary decisions, take into account both the general balance of your meals and their nutritional composition. You are certain to experience a multitude of health advantages when different nutrient-dense components are combined. For instance, a salad with almonds, berries, and mixed greens with a citrus dressing offers a meal that is high in fiber, good fats, and antioxidants. Eating a diet rich in whole grains, lean plant proteins, colorful vegetables, and fruits may provide a well-rounded approach to health maintenance and cancer prevention.

In summary, choosing foods high in fiber, phytonutrients, antioxidants, and healthy fats is a key component of utilizing nutritional information to influence your dietary decisions. Making better-educated choices about what to put in your diet may be achieved by being aware of the functions these nutrients play in preventing cancer and maintaining general health. A balanced and wholesome eating plan that promotes your well-being and fits with your dietary objectives may be made by including a variety of these essential items in your meals.

Resources for Further Reading

Many sites provide in-depth analyses and evidence-based recommendations for anyone who wants to learn more about a plant-based diet and its potential to prevent cancer. These resources include scholarly journals, books, and websites that provide regular updates on developments in the topic. They may support readers in staying informed and making well-informed dietary and health-related choices.

If you would rather go more into the topic of plant-based diet and how it affects cancer prevention, books are a great place to start. Dr. T. Colin Campbell and Thomas M. Campbell II's book "The China Study" comes highly recommended. The results of one of the largest studies on the connection between nutrition and illness are presented in this book, emphasizing the advantages of a plant-based diet in lowering the risk of cancer. Dr. Michael Greger's book "How Not to Die" is another noteworthy title. It focuses on the role that nutrition plays in preventing and treating chronic illnesses, such as cancer. For anybody interested in plant-based nutrition, Dr. Greger's practical counsel, grounded on the most recent scientific data, is a useful resource.

Academic journals and papers provide information on the topic that is supported by evidence and is peer-reviewed. Journals like "Nutrition and Cancer" and "The American Journal of Clinical Nutrition" often publish papers on nutrition and cancer for people who want to learn more about current research. These articles often provide insights into the most recent discoveries and current studies on the subject. Using internet databases or university libraries to access these articles may help readers remain current on research and advances.

Websites devoted to cancer prevention and plant-based diets provide a wide range of users with easily accessible and useful information. A plethora of information on nutrition and cancer prevention is available from the American Institute for Cancer Study (AICR), including dietary recommendations, study summaries, and nutritious recipe ideas. Their website is a wonderful resource for learning how certain food decisions might affect one's risk of cancer and general health. Dr. Michael Greger's NutritionFacts.org is another helpful resource. It offers articles and videos on a variety of nutrition-related and health-related subjects, such as cancer prevention and plant-based diets.

Participating in online forums and groups may help continue education. Active forums on plant-based diet and cancer prevention may be found on websites like Reddit, where people can ask questions, share personal stories, and debate the most recent findings. Furthermore, there is a constant supply of knowledge and inspiration on social media sites like Instagram and Twitter that include accounts and hashtags related to plant-based food and wellness.

Attending webinars, seminars, and conferences on nutrition and cancer prevention might help you expand your knowledge. Experts in the area address the most recent findings and trends in virtual events that are hosted by several organizations and institutions. These gatherings provide chances for hands-on education and networking with other people who have a love for plant-based diets.

Exploring these sites, analyzing the data critically, and keeping up with the most recent advancements are all part of continuing education on plant-based nutrition and cancer prevention. Readers may stay informed about how dietary decisions affect health and cancer risk by routinely reviewing reliable sources, taking part in educational activities, and interacting with educated communities. People are empowered to make choices and adopt habits that promote their well-being and illness prevention objectives via this continuous learning process.

Scan the QR Code or <u>Click Here</u> to get the book

Glossary of Terms

Understanding the terminology associated with plant-based nutrition and cancer prevention is crucial for effectively navigating dietary choices and making informed decisions about health. Familiarizing yourself with these key terms can help you better comprehend how specific ingredients and dietary practices contribute to overall well-being and cancer prevention.

Phytochemicals are naturally occurring compounds found in plant foods that have been shown to have health-promoting properties. These include antioxidants, which protect cells from damage caused by free radicals, and other compounds that can influence inflammation and immune function. Examples of phytochemicals include flavonoids found in berries and carotenoids found in carrots and sweet potatoes. Knowing about phytochemicals can help you identify foods that offer protective benefits.

Antioxidants are substances that help neutralize harmful free radicals in the body, thereby reducing oxidative stress and inflammation, which are linked to cancer development. Common antioxidants include vitamins C and E, selenium, and polyphenols. Understanding their role can guide you in choosing foods that are rich in these protective compounds.

Inflammation refers to the body's immune response to injury or infection. Chronic inflammation is linked to various diseases, including cancer. Foods with anti-inflammatory properties can help mitigate this risk. Ingredients such as turmeric, ginger, and omega-3 fatty acids found in flaxseeds and chia seeds are known for their anti-inflammatory effects. Recognizing these can assist you in incorporating more beneficial ingredients into your diet.

Glycemic Index (GI) measures how quickly a food raises blood sugar levels. Foods with a low glycemic index release glucose slowly into the bloodstream, helping to manage insulin levels and reduce cancer risk. Examples include legumes, whole grains, and non-starchy vegetables. Understanding GI can help you select foods that provide steady energy and support overall health.

Phytonutrients are compounds produced by plants that have beneficial effects on health. They include flavonoids, carotenoids, and glucosinolates, among others. Each type of phytonutrient has specific roles, such as supporting immune function or detoxifying the body. Learning about phytonutrients can guide you in choosing a variety of colorful fruits and vegetables to maximize their health benefits.

Omega-3 Fatty Acids are essential fats found in certain plant-based sources like flaxseeds, chia seeds, and walnuts. These fats play a crucial role in reducing inflammation and supporting heart health. Understanding their importance helps you include these sources in your diet for comprehensive health benefits.

Fiber is a type of carbohydrate that the body cannot digest, which aids in digestion and supports a healthy gut. High-fiber foods include whole grains, fruits, vegetables, and legumes. Fiber helps maintain regular bowel movements and may reduce the risk of colorectal cancer. Recognizing high-fiber foods ensures you incorporate them into your meals for digestive health.

Gluten-Free refers to foods that do not contain gluten, a protein found in wheat, barley, and rye. For individuals with celiac disease or gluten sensitivity, avoiding gluten is essential for health. Many plant-based foods, such as fruits, vegetables, and legumes, are naturally gluten-free, making them suitable options for those with dietary restrictions.

Complete Protein refers to proteins that contain all nine essential amino acids required by the body. While animal products are complete proteins, many plant-based sources, such as quinoa and soy products, also provide all essential amino acids. Understanding complete proteins helps ensure you get adequate protein from plant-based sources.

Detoxification is the process by which the body eliminates toxins. Certain plant-based foods, such as cruciferous vegetables and herbs like cilantro, support detoxification pathways in the liver and other organs. Knowledge of detoxifying foods can help you incorporate ingredients that aid in the body's natural cleansing processes.

Familiarity with these terms equips you with the knowledge to make informed decisions about your diet and health. By understanding how various ingredients and dietary practices contribute to cancer prevention and overall well-being, you can more effectively navigate your plant-based eating journey and optimize the benefits of your meals.

ACKNOWLEDGMENTS

This cookbook's creation has been an immensely fulfilling experience, made possible by the priceless contributions of many people and organizations. Their assistance, knowledge, and commitment have been crucial in making this project a success and guaranteeing its relevance and quality.

First and foremost, I would like to express my sincere appreciation to the nutritionists and culinary experts who offered their advice and insights throughout the recipe creation process. Their in-depth understanding of cancer prevention and plant-based nutrition proved invaluable in creating foods that are not only tasty but also in line with the most recent scientific findings. Their contributions guaranteed that every dish provides the required nutrients and health advantages, therefore establishing the cookbook as a dependable source for anyone looking to enhance their diet and overall health.

I express my sincere gratitude to the researchers and medical experts who examined the nutritional information and offered input on the advantages of different components for health. Their knowledge was useful in improving the recipes and making sure they met the strictest requirements for effectiveness and safety. Their willingness to work together and share their expertise has been crucial to the cookbook's success in being both practically helpful and scientifically correct.

We would especially want to thank the food stylists and photographers whose creative talents made the recipes come to life. The cookbook has visually captivating and motivating graphics that perfectly capture the spirit and charm of each meal. Their work inspires readers to try out the recipes and adopt a healthy lifestyle in addition to showcasing the beauty of plant-based food.

I also want to express my gratitude to the publishing team, whose expertise and assistance were crucial in turning my idea become a reality. Their proficiency in production, design, and editing made sure that the finished work was polished, unified, and easy to read. Their dedication to quality and meticulous attention to detail has been crucial to the cookbook's success.

We would also like to express our gratitude to all of the people who submitted their own experiences and tales. Their willingness to participate and be receptive to feedback has given the cookbook a more relevant and relatable human touch. Their experiences have served as inspiration for the development of nutrient-dense but specifically designed to meet the demands of cancer patients pursuing a plant-based diet.

I would be negligent if I did not thank my friends and family for their encouragement and input along the process. Their support of the endeavor and their helpful critiques were crucial in forming the finished product. Their encouragement kept me motivated to finish this task by serving as a regular reminder of its significance.

Lastly, a particular thank you to the institutions and organizations that support plant-based diets and the prevention of cancer. Their lobbying, educational initiatives, and research have served as a source of support and inspiration. Their contributions to the area have influenced the cookbook's content and bolstered its goal of equipping people with useful information and skills for improved health.

Each of these contributions has been instrumental in the development of this cookbook, and their combined efforts have produced an educational and useful resource. Their assistance has improved the content's quality and given readers a better overall experience. Their commitment and knowledge are evident in this cookbook, and I am very appreciative of what they contributed.

ABOUT THE AUTHOR

Kelley Hamilton is a singular voice in the world of nutrition and cancer prevention because of her extensive knowledge and personal touch. Kelley has devoted her professional life to investigating the complex relationships between nutrition, lifestyle, and illness management because she has a strong enthusiasm for health and well-being. Her upbringing and life experiences have influenced her methodology and given her work a genuine and compassionate quality.

A solid foundation in nutrition science and health education forms the basis of Kelley's academic career. Her graduate degrees are in dietetics and nutrition, with an emphasis on managing and preventing cancer. Her research has given her a thorough grasp of how various dietary patterns affect general health and, in particular, how to use them to help cancer patients. Her practical experience working in clinical settings, where she has utilized her expertise to help patients in adopting nutritional changes that support their treatment and recovery, complements her academic brilliance.

Her career path has been distinguished by her steadfast adherence to evidence-based practice and her constant pursuit of the most recent advancements in the field of nutrition science. Kelley has developed and implemented dietary programs that are in line with best practices and current scientific knowledge in close collaboration with healthcare professionals. Her abilities have improved as a result of this experience, and it has also strengthened her conviction that nutrition plays a crucial role in managing and preventing cancer.

Kelley has a very individualized approach to eating that is influenced by her struggles and experiences. She is aware of the psychological and physical toll that a cancer diagnosis can have since she has personally handled the difficulties of receiving a diagnosis in her own family. Her work has a distinct viewpoint because of her connection to the topic. It motivates her to create useful, scientifically based tools that inspire and help those going through comparable struggles.

This cookbook's methodology and content are a clear representation of Kelley's career experience and life experiences. Every dish is created to offer comfort and enjoyment in addition to nutritional value. Kelley's emphasis on a plant-based diet stems from her conviction that it can improve health outcomes. She has carefully chosen ingredients and created delectable dishes that are in line with the most recent findings on cancer treatment and prevention.

Apart from her academic credentials, Kelley has a strong belief in empowering others with knowledge and useful resources. To encourage better eating habits, she has engaged communities and shared her experience by conducting workshops and seminars. Her method, which combines discipline and compassion, aims to inform and encourage people who want to make better food choices to enhance their health.

There is more to Kelley's commitment to this endeavor than what is written in the cookbook. She is dedicated to lifelong learning and research, always looking for fresh data and perspectives that might improve the efficacy of her suggestions. Her commitment to personal development and her involvement in the larger community guarantee that her work will always be significant and relevant.

In addition to recipes, Kelley Hamilton provides a comprehensive strategy for health and wellbeing in her cookbook. Her upbringing and life events have molded her into a resource that is profoundly compassionate and anchored in science. Her work is an invaluable resource for anybody wishing to incorporate plant-based nutrition into their life, especially those who are managing cancer or trying to avoid it, due to her unique combination of knowledge and personal understanding.

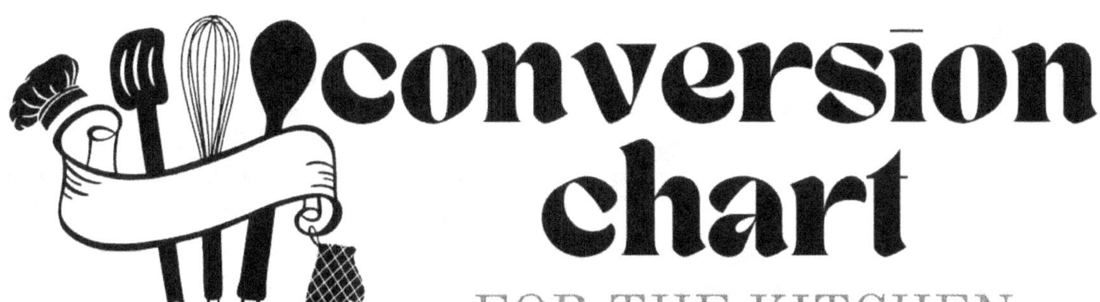

VOLUME MEASUREMENT CONVERSIONS

Cups	Tablespoons	Teaspoons	Milliliters
1/16 cup	1 tbsp	1 tsp	5ml
1/8 cup	2 tbsp	3 tsp	15 ml
1/4 cup	4 tbsp	6 tsp	30 ml
1/3 cup	5 1/3 tbsp	12 tsp	60 ml
1/2 cup	8 tbsp	16 tsp	80 ml
2/3 cup	10 2/3 tbsp	24 tsp	120 ml
3/4 cup	12 tbsp	32 tsp	160 ml
1 cup	16 tbsp	36 tsp	180 ml
		48 tsp	240 ml

1 QUART =
2 pints
4 cups
32 ounces
950 ml

1 PINT =
2 cups
16 ounces
480 ml

1 CUP =
16tbsp
8 ounces
240 ml

1/4 CUP =
4 tbsp
12 tsp
2 ounces
60 ml

1 TBSP =
3 tsp 1/2
ounce
15 ml

COOKING TEMPERATURE CONVERSIONS

Celcius/Centigrade $\quad F = (C \times 1.8) + 32$

Fahrenheit $\quad C = (F - 32) \times 0.5556$

BAKING INGREDIENT CONVERSIONS

BUTTER

Cups	Grams
1/4 cup	57 grams
1/3 cup	76 grams
1/2 cup	113 grams
1 cup	227 grams

PACKED BROWN SUGAR

Cups	Grams	Ounces
1/4 cup	55 grams	1.9 oz
1/3 cup	73 grams	2.58 oz
1/2 cup	110 grams	3.88 oz
1 cup	220 grams	7.75 oz

ALL-PURPOSE FLOUR / CONFECTIONER'S SUGAR

Cups	Grams	Ounces
1/8 cup	16 grams	563 oz
1/4 cup	32 grams	1.13 oz
1/3 cup	43 grams	1.5 oz
1/2 cup	64 grams	2.25 oz
2/3 cup	85 grams	3 oz
3/4 cup	96 grams	3.38 oz
1 cup	128 grams	4.5 oz

GRANULATED SUGAR

Cups	Grams	Ounces
2 tbsp	25 grams	89 oz
1/4 cup	67 grams	1.78 oz
1/3 cup	50 grams	2.37 oz
1/2 cup	100 grams	3.55 oz
2/3 cup	134 grams	4.73 oz
3/4 cup	150 grams	5.3 oz
1 cup	201 grams	7.1 oz

MONDAY

__ / __ / ____

TRACK TODAY

	BEFORE	AFTER
BREAK FAST		
LUNCH		
SNACK		
DINNER		

NOTE

MOOD:

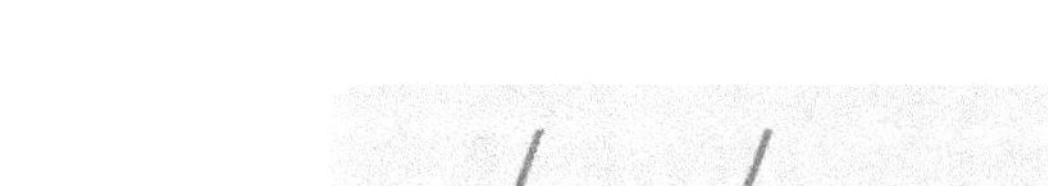

TUESDAY

__ / __ / ____

TRACK TODAY

	BEFORE	AFTER
BREAK FAST		
LUNCH		
SNACK		
DINNER		

NOTE

MOOD:

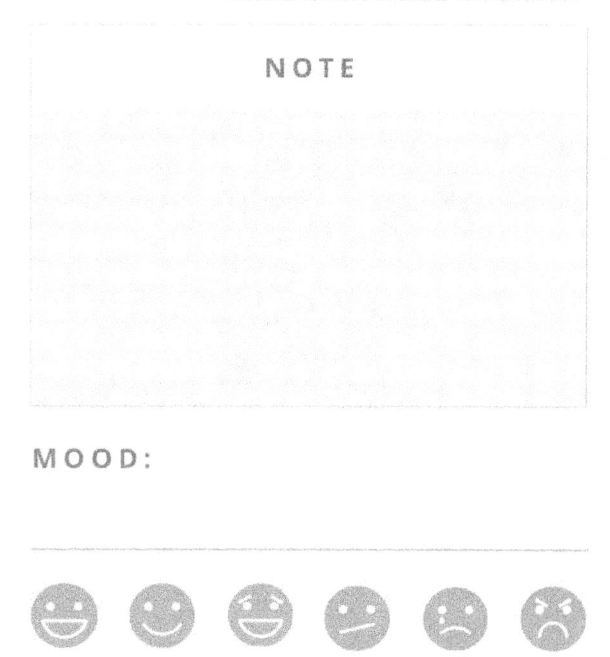

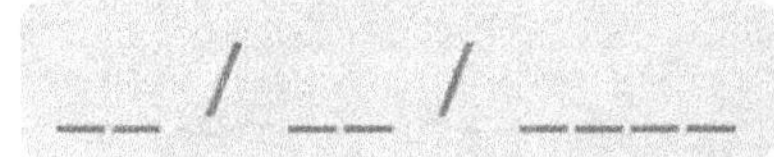

__ / __ / ____

	BEFORE	AFTER
TRACK TODAY		
BREAK FAST		
LUNCH		
SNACK		
DINNER		

NOTE:

MOOD:

THURSDAY

__ / __ / ____

	BEFORE	AFTER
TRACK TODAY		
BREAK FAST		
LUNCH		
SNACK		
DINNER		

NOTE:

MOOD:

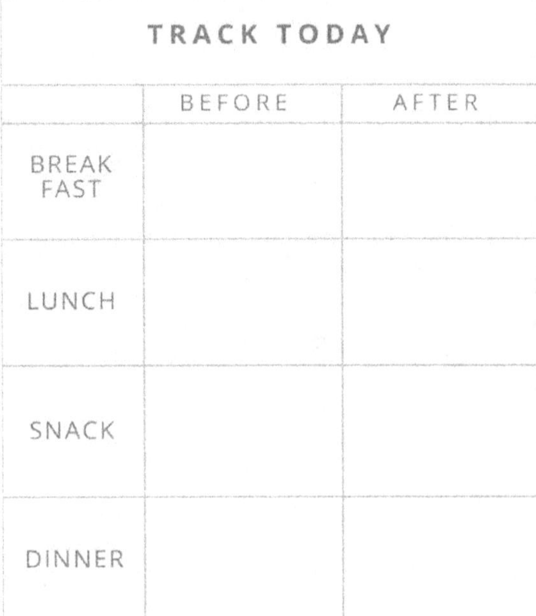

FRIDAY

TRACK TODAY

	BEFORE	AFTER
BREAK FAST		
LUNCH		
SNACK		
DINNER		

NOTE:

MOOD:

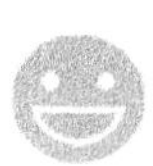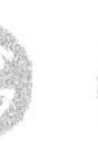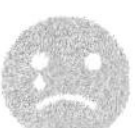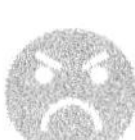
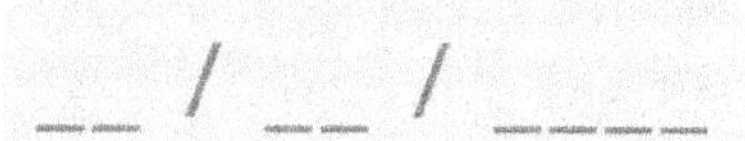

SATURDAY

TRACK TODAY

	BEFORE	AFTER
BREAK FAST		
LUNCH		
SNACK		
DINNER		

NOTE:

MOOD:

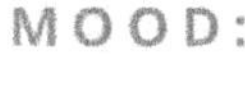
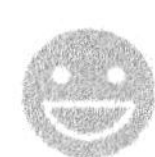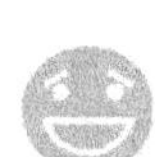

SUNDAY

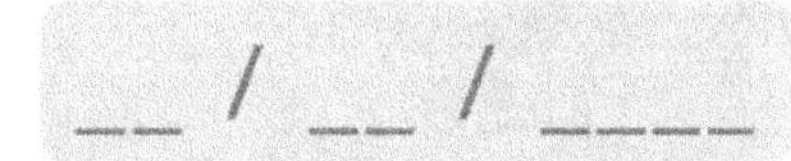

TRACK TODAY

	BEFORE	AFTER
BREAK FAST		
LUNCH		
SNACK		
DINNER		

NOTE:

MOOD:

WEEKLY SUMMARY